AF556720

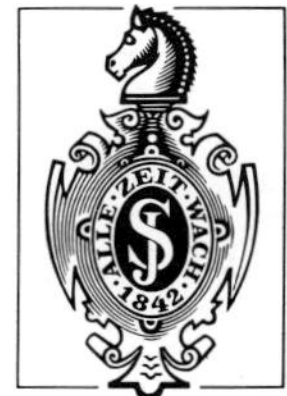
ALLE · ZEIT · WACH
1842

Manuel Viamonte Jr.

Errors in Uroradiology

With 148 Figures (41 Cases)
in 173 Separate Illustrations

Springer-Verlag
Berlin Heidelberg New York
London Paris Tokyo
Hong Kong Barcelona
Budapest

Prof. Manuel Viamonte Jr., M.D., M.Sc.
Chairman and Director
Department of Radiology
Mount Sinai Medical Center
Prof. of Radiology
University of Miami School of Medicine
4300 Alton Road
Miami Beach, FL 33140
USA

ISBN 3-540-54504-2 Springer-Verlag Berlin Heidelberg New York
ISBN 0-387-54504-2 Springer-Verlag New York Berlin Heidelberg

Library of Congress Cataloging-in-Publication Data. Viamonte, Manuel, 1930 –. Errors in uroradiology / Manuel Viamonte Jr., p. cm.
ISBN 3-540-54504-2 (Berlin). – ISBN 0-387-54504-2 (New York)
1. Urinary organs–Radiography. 2. Diagnostic errors. I. Title.
RC874.V53 1992 616.6′07572–dc20 92-10890 CIP

Reproduction of the figures: Gustav Dreher GmbH, Stuttgart, FRG
Typesetting, printing and binding: Konrad Triltsch, Graphischer Betrieb, Würzburg, FRG
21/3130-5 4 3 2 1 0 – Printed on acid-free paper

The most fruitful lesson is the conquest of one's own error. Whoever refuses to admit error may be a great scholar but he is not a great learner. Whoever is ashamed of error will struggle against recognizing and admitting it, which means that he struggles against his greatest inward gain.

J. W. v. Goethe, *Maxims and Reflections*

Acknowledgements

Grateful acknowledgement is given to the following for permission to use of figures in this publication:

Williams and Wilkins Company for figures from Viamonte M Jr, Ravel R, Politano V, Bridges B (1976) Angiographic findings in a patient with tuberous sclerosis. Am J Roentgenol 98: 723

Radiological Society of North America for figures from Zeman RK, Cronan JJ, Rosenfeld T et al. (1986) Computed tomography of renal masses: pitfalls and anatomic variants. Radiographics 6: 351–372

Cahners Publishing Company (Urology) for figures from Viamonte M, Viamonte M Jr, Rywlin A, Roen S, Casal G (1980) Subepithelial hemorrhage of renal pelvis simulating neoplasm (Antopol-Goldman lesion). Urology 16

Harold Batt, M.D., University of Miami School of Medicine, Miami, FL, USA, for cases 7–11 and 49

Contents

Introduction

This monograph deals primarily with the kidneys, ureters, and urinary bladder.

The kidneys are retroperitoneal structures that parallel the psoas muscle. The left kidney is usually slightly higher than the right and is slightly more medially located. The vertical axis of the kidneys, when compared with the midline, is about 20°. There is often considerable mobility of the kidneys as a result of respiration and body position. Several centimeters of excursion have been demonstrated on deep inspiration or in the upright position.

During late embryological development, each kidney occupies the flank region, capped by the liver on the right side and the spleen on the left. Abnormalities of the liver and spleen can affect the position of the kidneys. Also, retroperitoneal masses may displace the kidney. A palpable abdominal mass which radiographically may appear to be an intraperitoneal structure can be accurately localized as a retroperitoneal tumor by observing displacement of the kidney, particularly if the kidney is pushed caudally and medially, superiorly and laterally, or medially.

Anomalies of the kidneys include abnormal position, abnormal number, changes in shape, and alterations in the inner structure that may affect the renal parenchyma, the pelvocalyceal systems, or both.

Abnormalities in kidney position range from simple malrotation (failure of rotation of the kidney along its vertical axis) to abnormal location of the kidney (renal ectopia). The incidence of renal ectopia varies from 1 in 500 to 1 in 1200. The most common form of ectopia is the pelvic kidney; in this condition the kidneys are located either in the true pelvis or at the pelvic inlet (abdominal ectopia). Other than the presence of a "pelvic mass," patients with pelvic kidney may have pain related to obstruction or infection and symptoms that may be attributable to a gastrointestinal disorder. Obstruction of the ureteropelvic junction, cryptorchidism, hypospadias in the male, vaginal agenesis, and extraurinary anomalies [vertebral and rib abnormalities, septal defects, and gastrointestinal tract anomalies (malrotation, perforated anus, etc.)] may be present. It has been reported that in about 50% of patients with unilateral renal ectopia an abnormality of the normally positioned kidney will also be present. During pregnancy, compression of ureters and kidneys with resulting infection and renal failure may occur. Likewise, in patients with horseshoe kidneys, compression of ureters trapped between the enlarging uterus and the tandem kidneys can lead to hydronephrosis, infection, and renal insufficiency. With renal agenesis (which occurs in 1 in 500 to 1 in 1500 births) and with renal ectopia, bowel and pancreatic relocation may occur.

Following nephrectomies, organ relocation also can be expected. Absence of the right kidney can simulate a right paraduodenal hernia. Absence of the left kidney can simulate a left flank tumor by virtue of the dorsally relocated tail of the pancreas.

When kidneys are in an abnormal position, their shape may change. The coffee-bean shape is seen almost exclusively with normally placed kidneys. Ectopic kidneys usually have an abnormal shape. Masses in malformed kidneys may represent carcinoma. I recommend periodic ultrasonography to establish early the appearance of a carcinoma.

Radiological Techniques

Plain radiography remains the initial screening technique for the retroperitoneum. It should be employed to visualize the outline of the liver, spleen, and kidneys, the fat-muscle interfaces of the psoas and pelvic muscles, and the position of the stomach and bowel (small and large); it also permits analysis of the spine and the supradiaphragmatic and inguinal regions. Only after due consideration has been given to these aspects may any further evaluation of the urinary tract be performed.

The presence of calcification(s) and the possibility of a fatty mass should be ruled out. When the appearance is suggestive of calcifications, one should consider the possibility that it is in fact due to opaque medication or a foreign body. Large calculi in the urinary bladder can simulate injected contrast material (following cystography). Calcific densities in the pelvis may be located in the alimentary tract, the pelvic vessels, or the pelvic lymph nodes; in the alimentary tract they may be the result of calcified fat, stones, or medication.

In addition to reviewing the patient's clinical history one should always check their eating habits and ask about medications. If calcific densities are present, it is important to ascertain whether any interventional examinations have been performed, such as retrograde pyelography. Retrograde pyelography should be used not as a primary diagnostic method but only as an adjunctive technique when standard procedures fail to demonstrate suspected pathology.

Antegrade pyelography is performed primarily for percutaneous nephrostomy and other interventional procedures, or for some urodynamic studies.

Cystography, urethrography, cavernosography, and vasography are additional contrast studies that have specific indications and limitations.

Excretory urography requires the use of radiopaque contrast material, usually injected into a peripheral vein. Excretory urography is a tailored examination that should take into consideration the reasons for the study, the clinical condition of the patient, and the possibility of contraindications for the injection of contrast material. The radiographic examination should include standard tomography, best obtained in the frontal and oblique projections. Particularly in elderly patients, where bowel preparation is often not present, and in patients with poor renal function, tomography will compensate to a reasonable degree and show the outline of the kidneys and the pelvocalyceal system.

In addition to supine films, obliques, prone views, and compression films should be used judiciously. A film of the abdomen should always be obtained upon completion of an angiographic study in order to evaluate kidney size, shape, position, and function and to detect unsuspected pathology. When angiocardiograms are performed in patients with congenital heart disease, a large number of associated renal anomalies that are clinically unsuspected are found.

Ultrasonography supplemented by the Doppler technique is the most popular noninvasive screening method for assessment of the kidneys. It enables one to examine the architecture of the kidney, to diagnose vascular abnormalities, to differentiate cystic from solid masses, to assess hydronephrosis, and to determine the resistive index. Ultrasonography of the bladder, prostate, seminal vesicle, and scrotum is of great value.

The second most important noninvasive imaging modality is *computed tomography* (CT). It has been possible with CT to detect minute lesions. CT is not a true screening technique as it requires injection of contrast material. It is more expensive and more time-consuming than ultrasonography. However, it is the best radiographic modality we have at this time to assess the renal parenchyma.

Magnetic resonance imaging (MRI) does not use ionizing radiation and provides multiplanar acquisition images and superb contrast resolution. It can establish the presence of patency of major vessels and of clots and tumors in the renal veins and/or the inferior vena cava. MRI competes with CT in the study of solid parenchymal organs. Because it is more expensive and not as readily available, it is not at present used as extensively as ultrasonography and CT.

Radionuclide Studies. Renal blood flow analysis, renal imaging, and renal function studies are valuable. They supplement information obtained using other noninvasive imaging modalities such as ultrasonography and CT.

Invasive Techniques. Angiography (arteriography, venography, and lymphography) has been utilized less frequently since the advent of noninvasive imaging modalities. Arterial studies can be used for therapeutic as well as for diagnostic purposes. Percutaneous biopsies, puncture of renal masses (i.e., diagnostic and therapeutic puncture of renal cysts), and other invasive procedures (i.e., angioplasty, stent placement) complete the state-of-the-art radiological armamentarium for the evaluation of the kidneys.

Format of This Book

This book highlights the more frequent sources of error when interpreting urograms and uroradiologic images obtained with other procedures. The book is accordingly divided into a number of sections, and as an aid to the reader the relevant section heading appears at the top of each page. Whenever a case number appears in a figure legend, the illustrations relate specifically to a case that either gave rise to error or represented a potential source of error. In addition a number of figures are included simply to illustrate characteristic clinical or radiologic features of certain entities, cognizance of which is invaluable in avoiding unnecessary errors.

Renal parenchymal hypertrophy may be of developmental origin (fetal lobulation, polar hypertrophy, thickened column of Bertin) or may be acquired (compensatory hypertrophy) secondary to inflammatory disease (i.e., pyelonephritis), infarction, or partial nephrectomy.

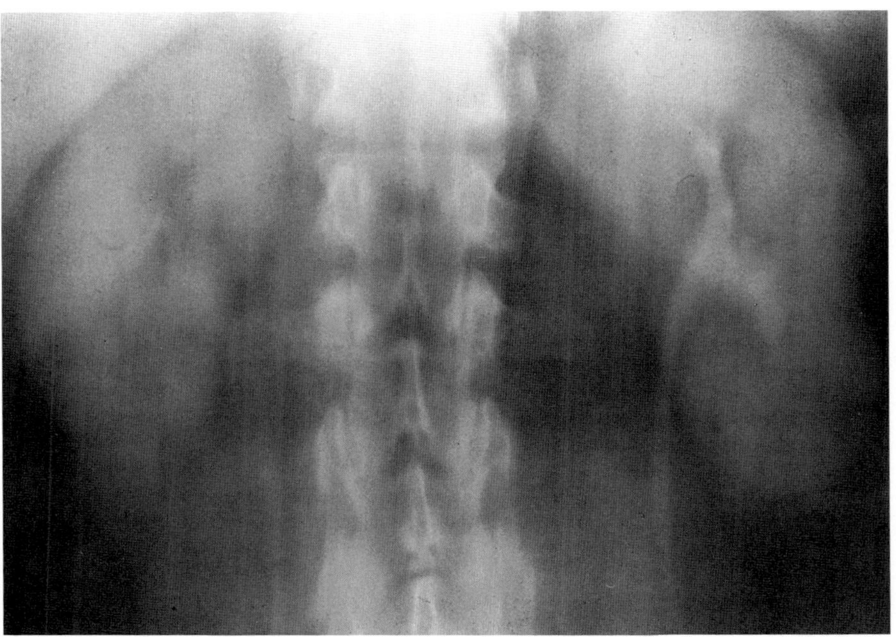

Fig. 1. Case 1. Excretory urogram showing a prominent upper pole of the left kidney

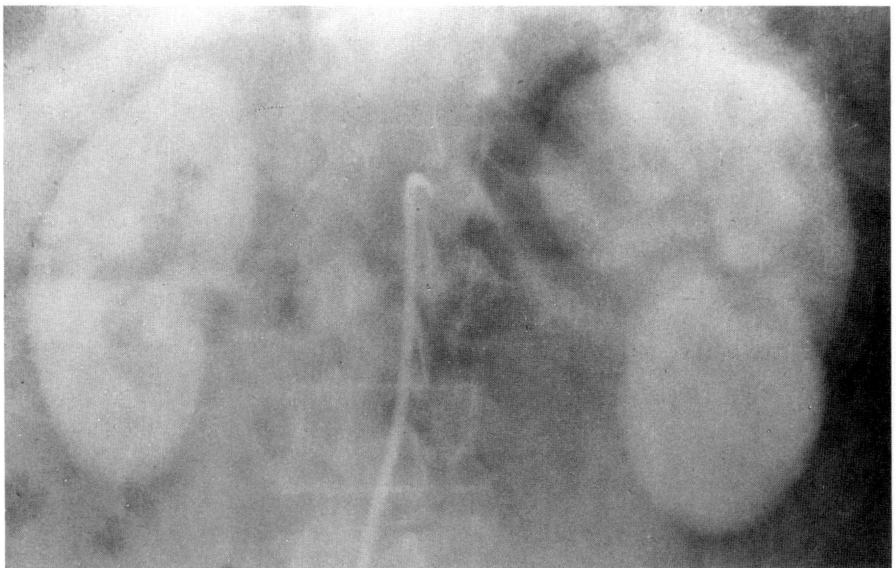

Fig. 2. Case 1. Late phase of an angiogram showing uniform density of the upper pole and a nodular density in the central portion of the left kidney. The former was related to polar hypertrophy and the latter to an area of cortical invagination (prominent column of Bertin)

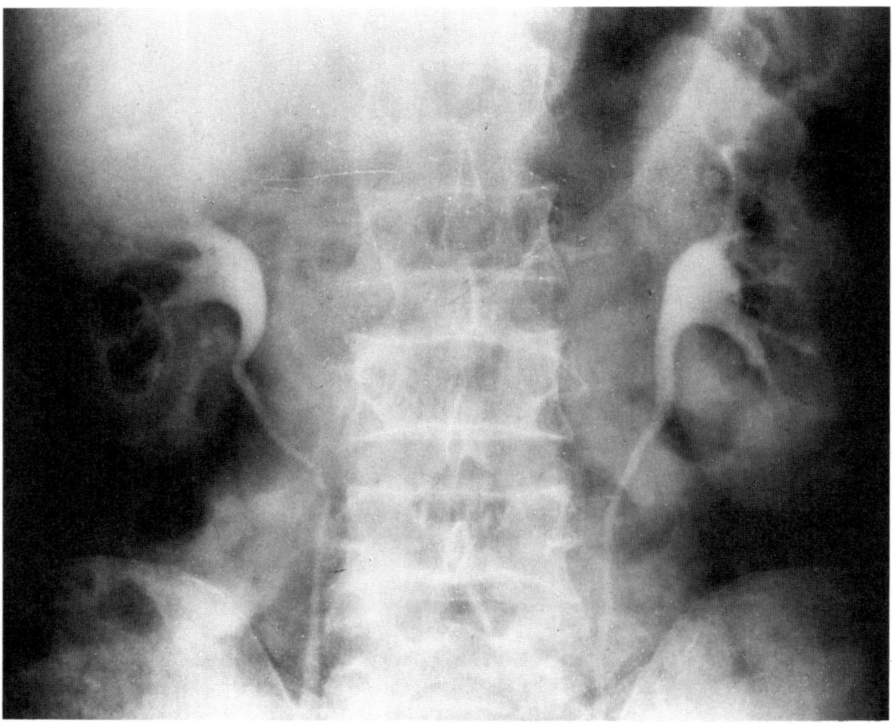

Fig. 3. Case 2. Excretory urogram showing prominence of the upper pole of the right kidney. Note elongation of the right upper infundibulum. These two findings suggested the possibility of a neoplasm. The patient was asymptomatic

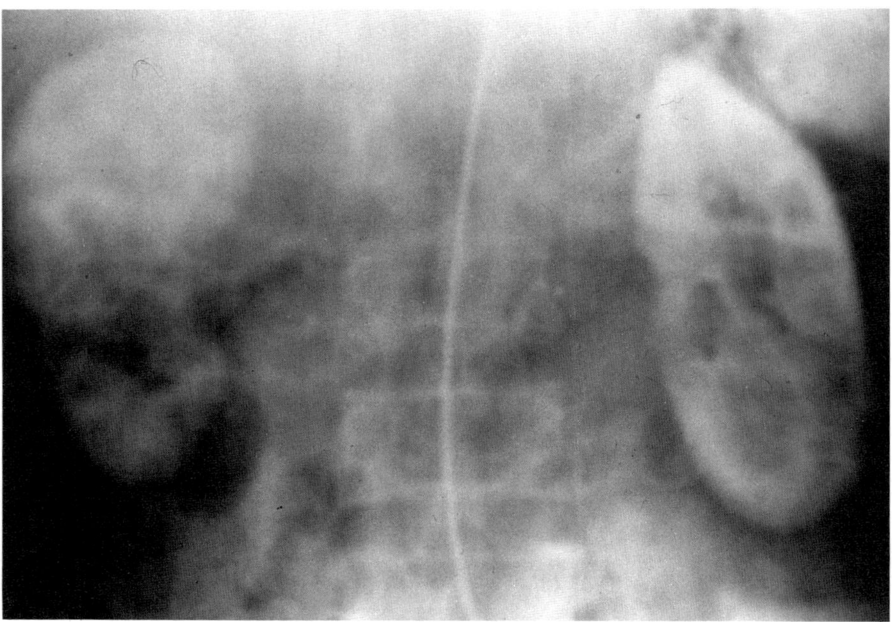

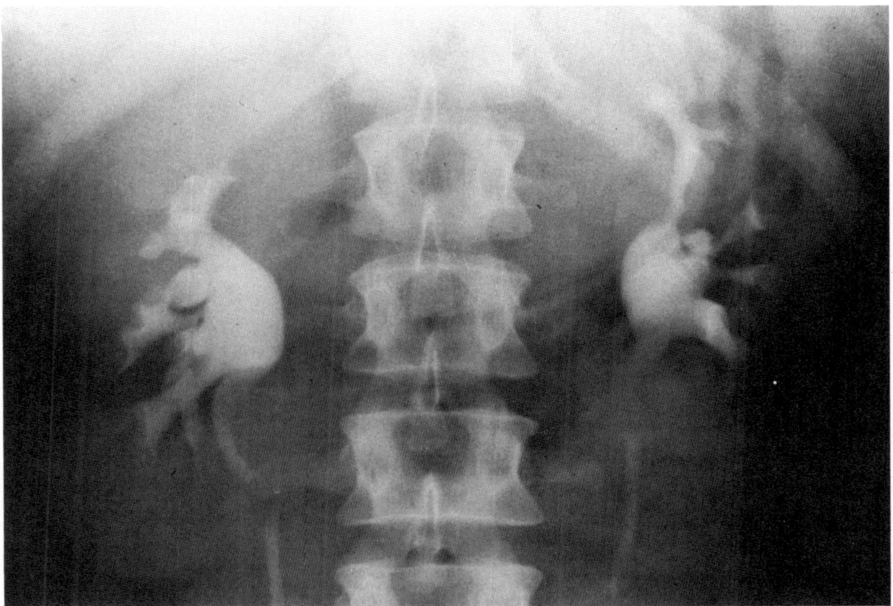

Fig. 5. Case 3. Excretory urogram showing the upper urinary tract in a patient who presented with lower urinary tract problems. Note mass in the lower pole of the right kidney with lateral displacement of the proximal right ureter

Fig. 4. Case 2. Late phase of an angiogram. Again, note uniform opacification of the upper pole of the right kidney. Biopsy showed no evidence of a tumor

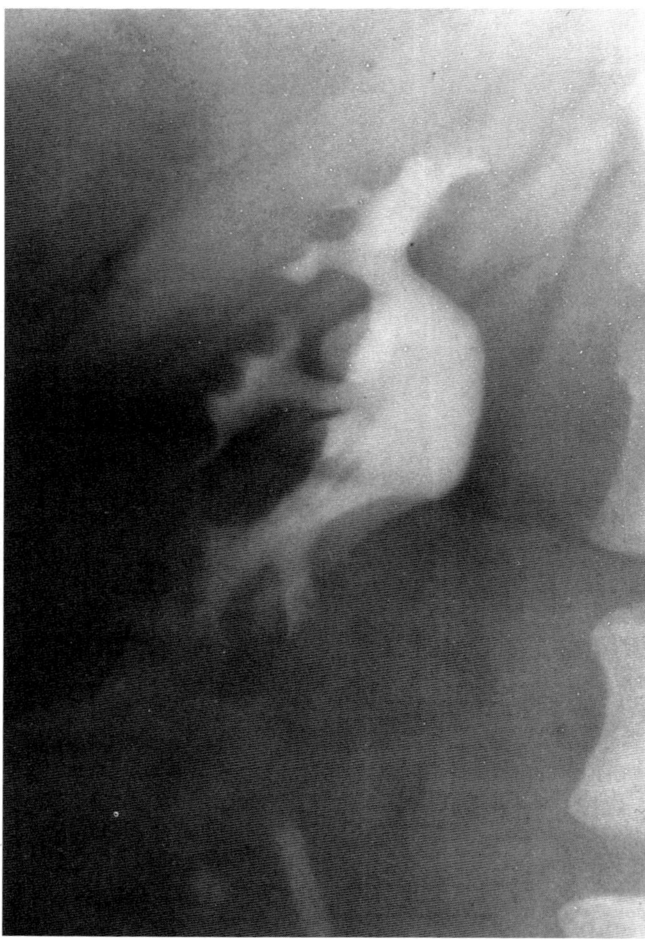

Fig. 6. Case 3. Right posterior oblique view of the right kidney showing mass in the lower pole, compression of the lower aspect of the right renal pelvis, and displacement of the right ureter laterally

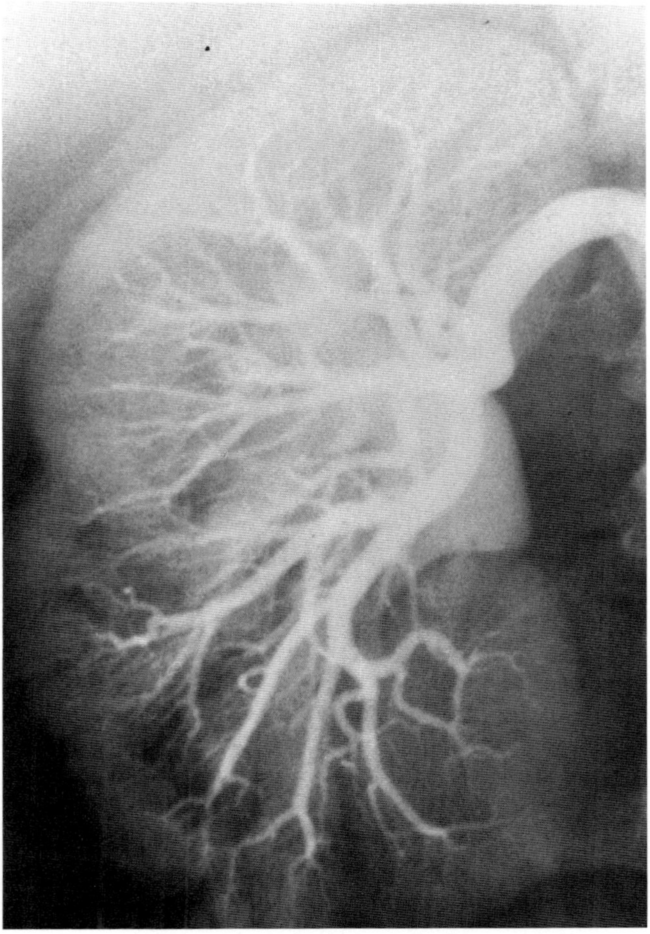

Fig. 7. Case 3. Right renal arteriogram, early arterial phase, showing normal arteries to the hypertrophied lower pole of the right kidney

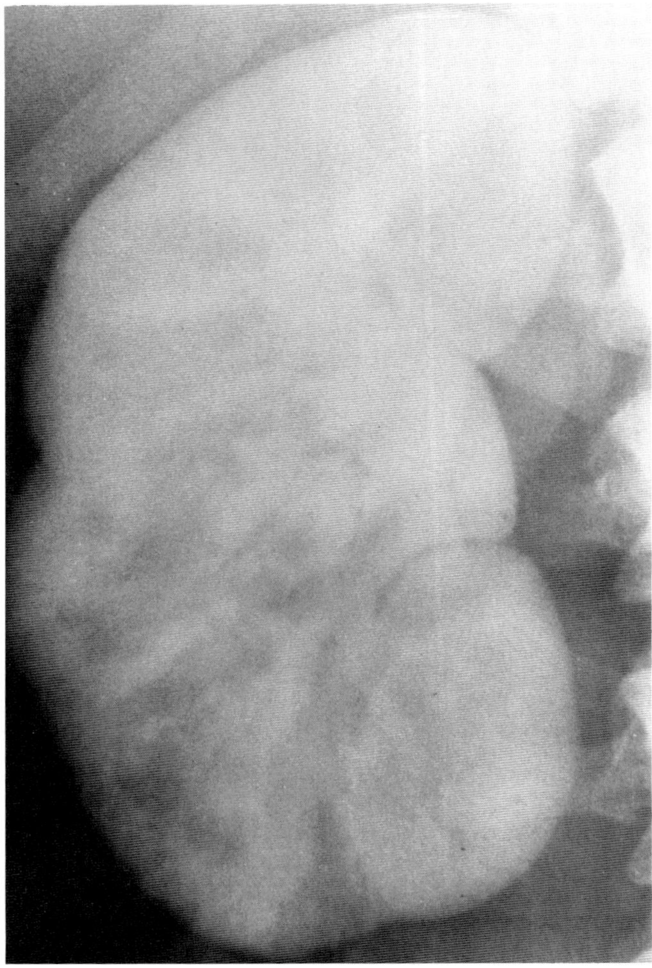

Fig. 8. Case 3. Right renal arteriogram, parenchymal phase, showing hypertrophy of the lower pole with fetal lobulation. There was no evidence of a tumor

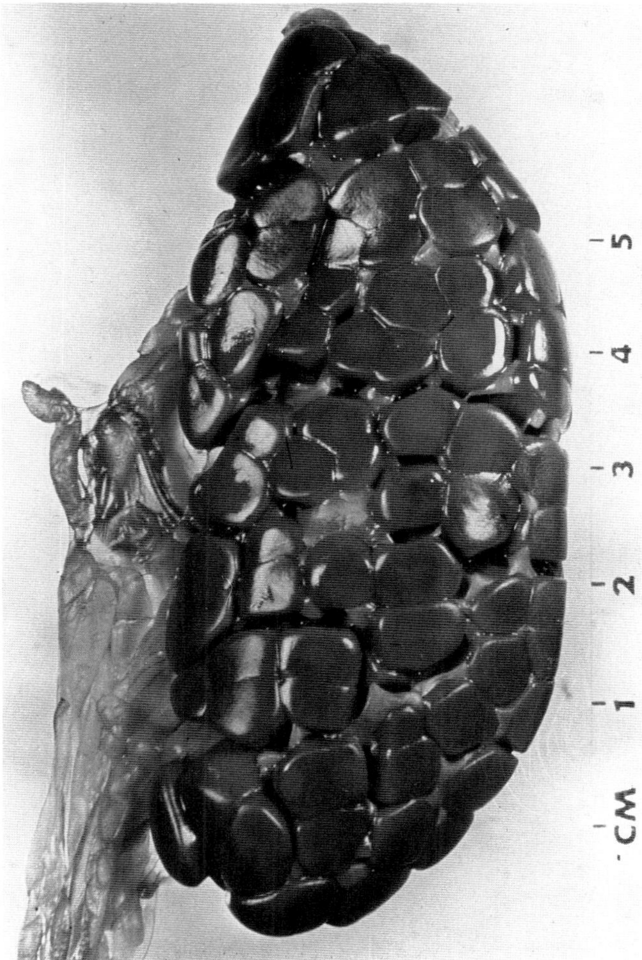

Fig. 9. Kidney of an adult sea otter. Note lobular surface (reniculi). During embryological development of a human kidney similar lobulations are found. When several fail to fuse, persistent fetal lobulations can mimic a renal mass

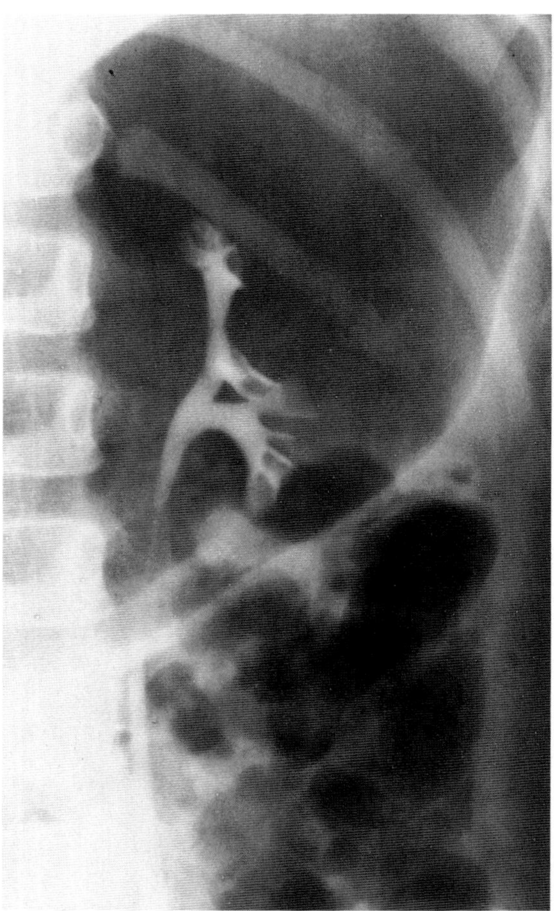

Fig. 10. Case 4. Close-up of the left kidney showing compression and displacement of the left middle calyx

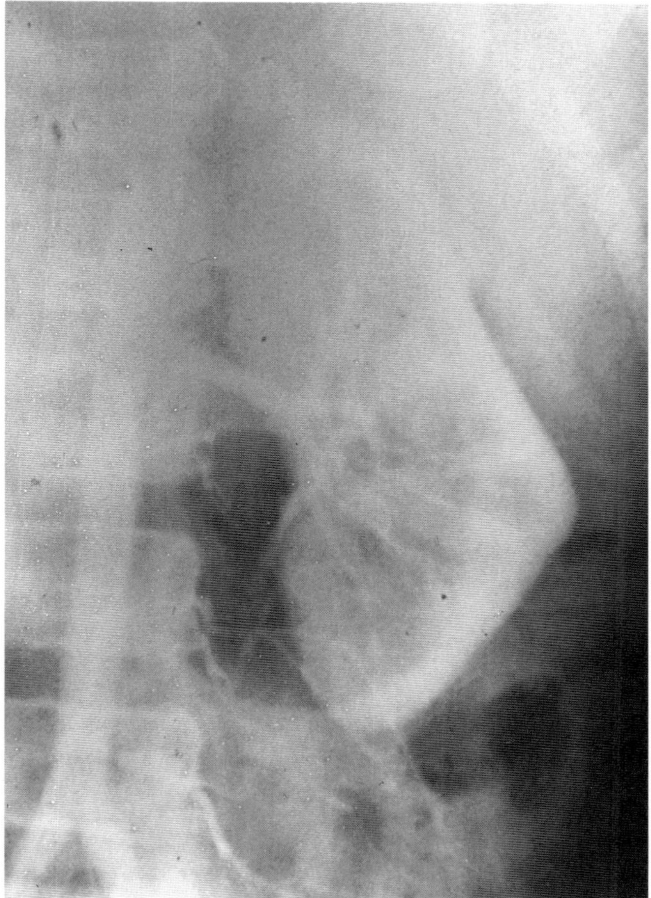

Fig. 11. Case 4. Aortogram, early arterial phase. Note density in the central portion of the left kidney close to the left middle calyx. This was interpreted as a neoplasm. The left kidney was removed

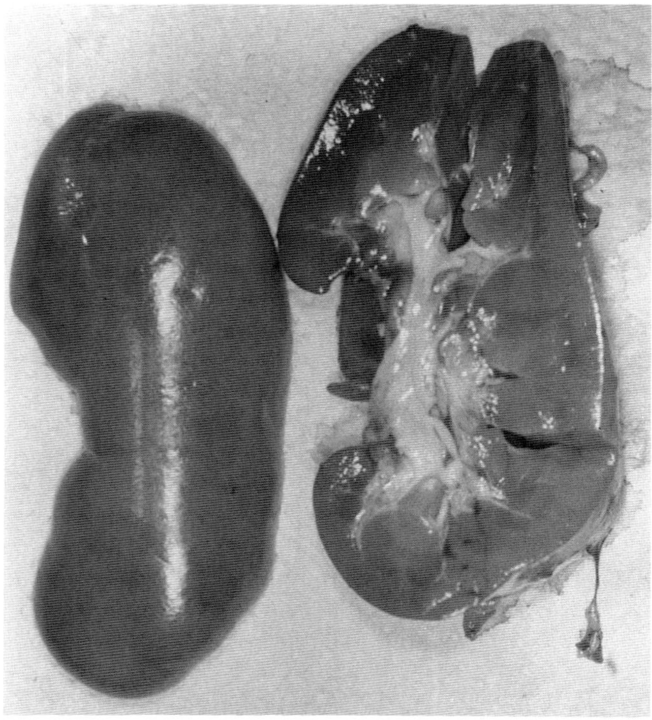

Fig. 12. Case 4. Cut specimen reveals parenchymal hypertrophy and cortical invagination simulating a neoplasm. No tumor was found histologically

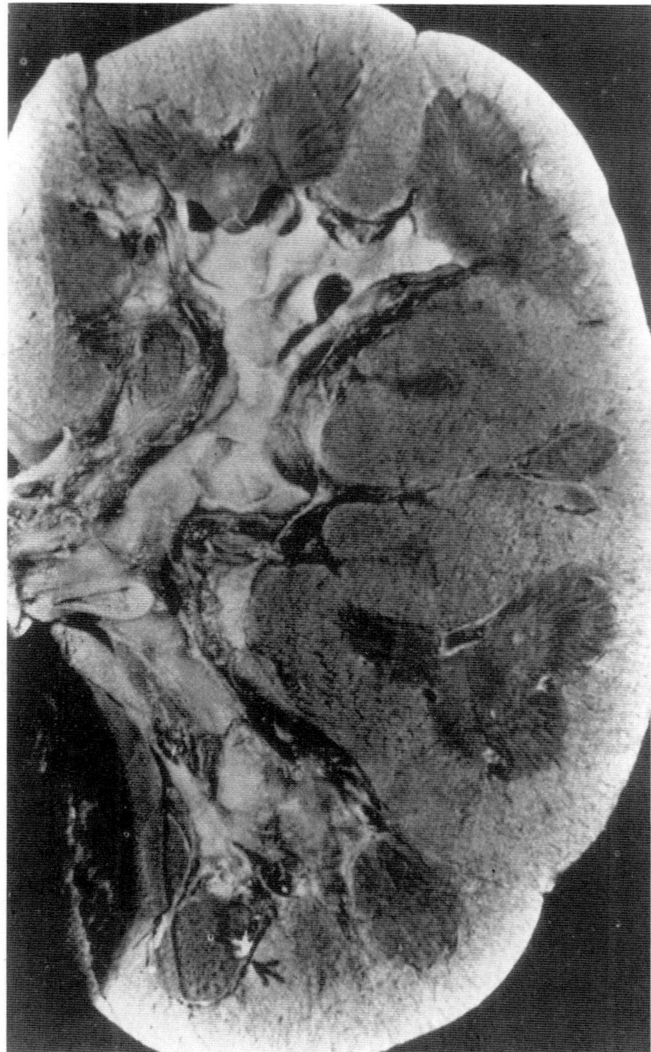

Fig. 13. Case 5. Coronal section of a kidney showing invagination of the cortex. This entity has also been called renal dysmorphism, cloisson by Hudson, or cortical invagination

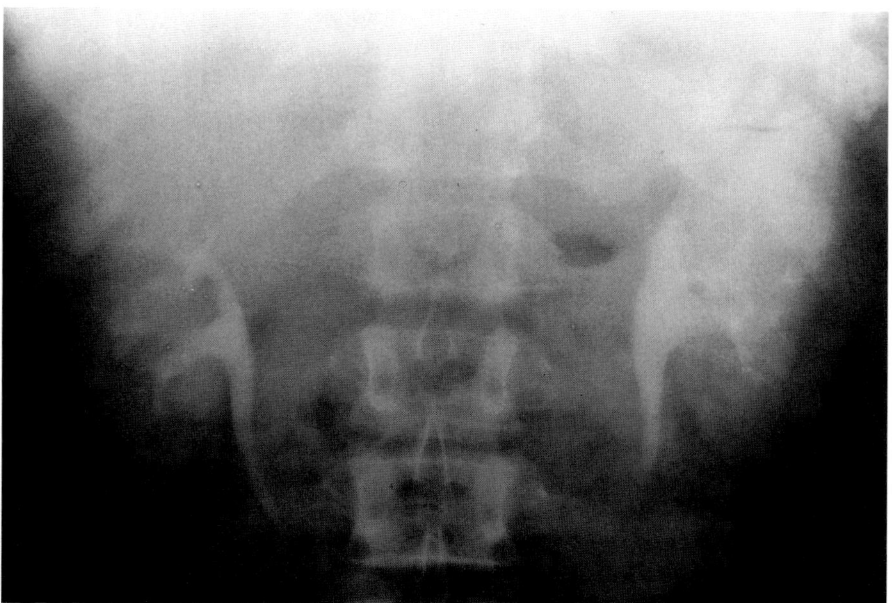

Fig. 14. Case 6. Excretory urogram in a patient with hematuria. The upper urinary tract shows a hypoplastic left middle calyx and a mass effect in the central portion of the left kidney

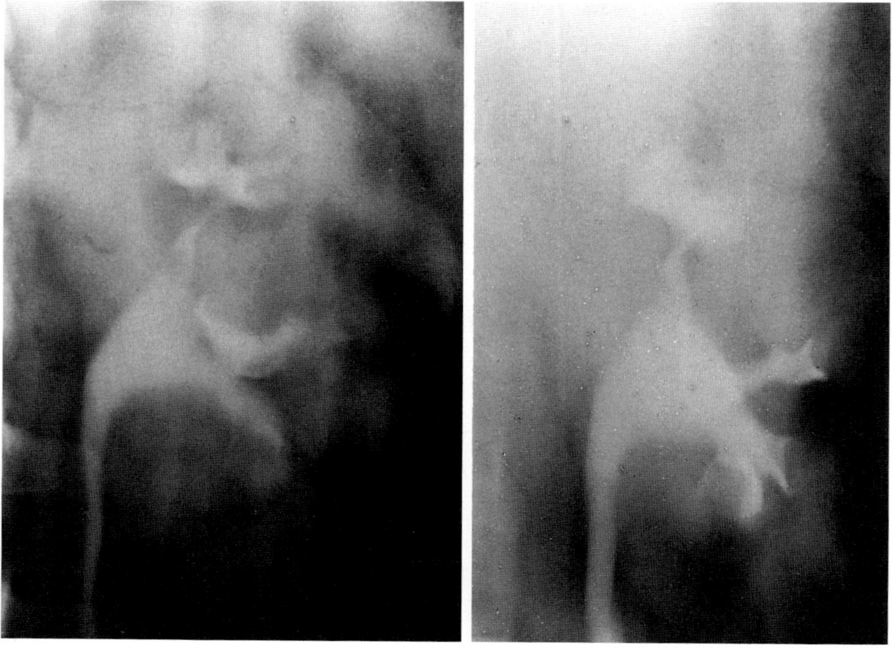

a b

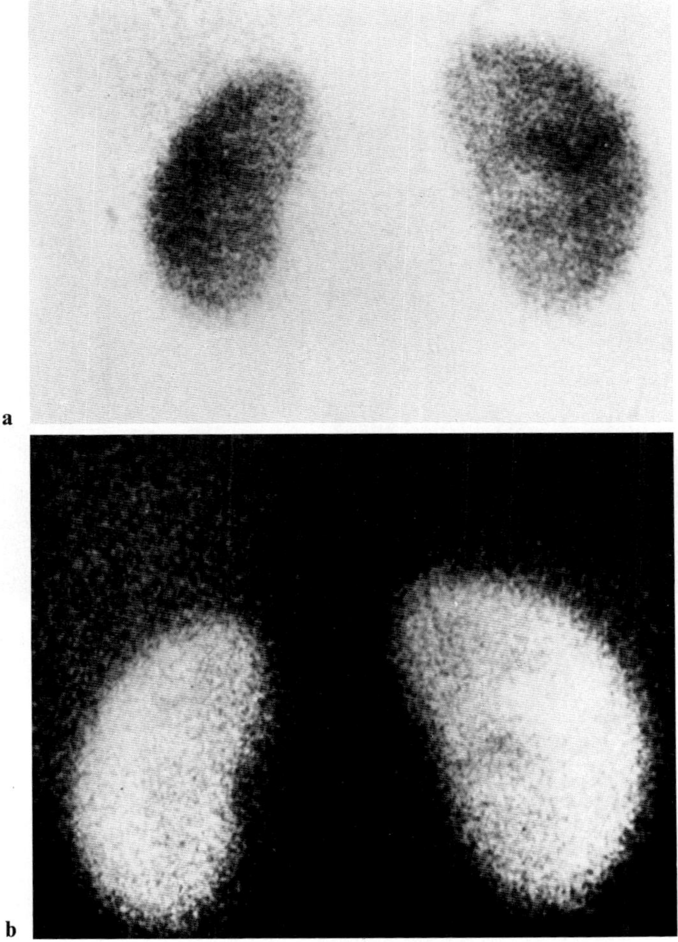

Fig. 16a, b. Case 6. Isotopic study showing intense activity in the central portion of the left kidney. This is pathognomonic of parenchymal hypertrophy. No tumor was present

Fig. 15a, b. Case 6. Tomographic sections revealing the compression and downward displacement of the left middle calyx

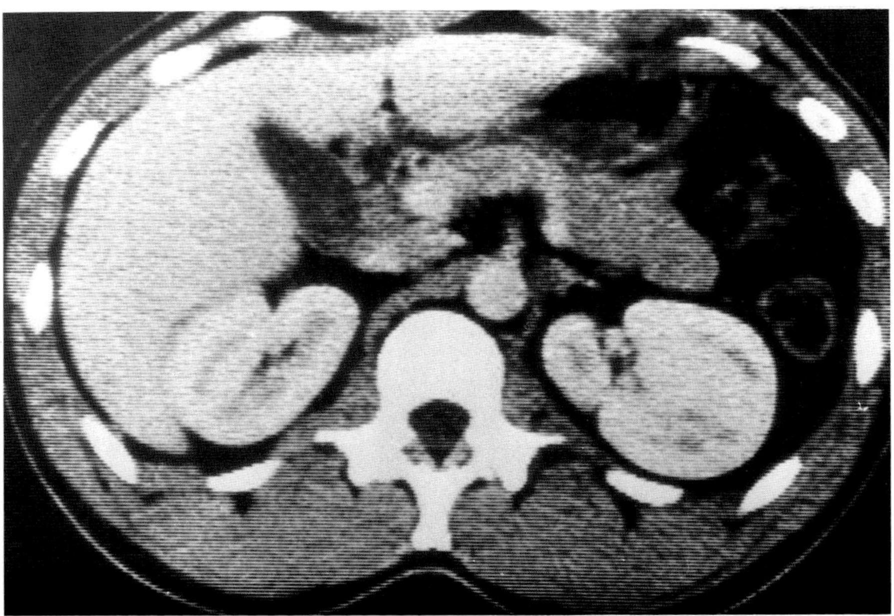

Fig. 17. Case 6. CT scan showing invagination of the cortex in the central portion of the left kidney

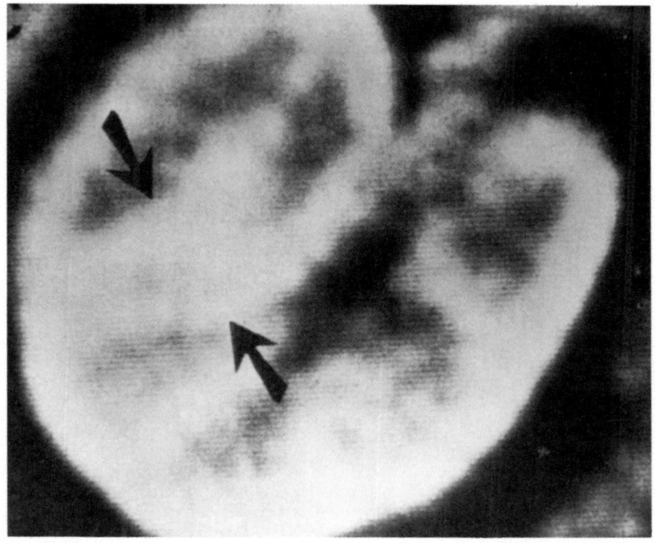

Fig. 18. Case 7. Prominent column of Bertin (*arrows*) in a CT examination

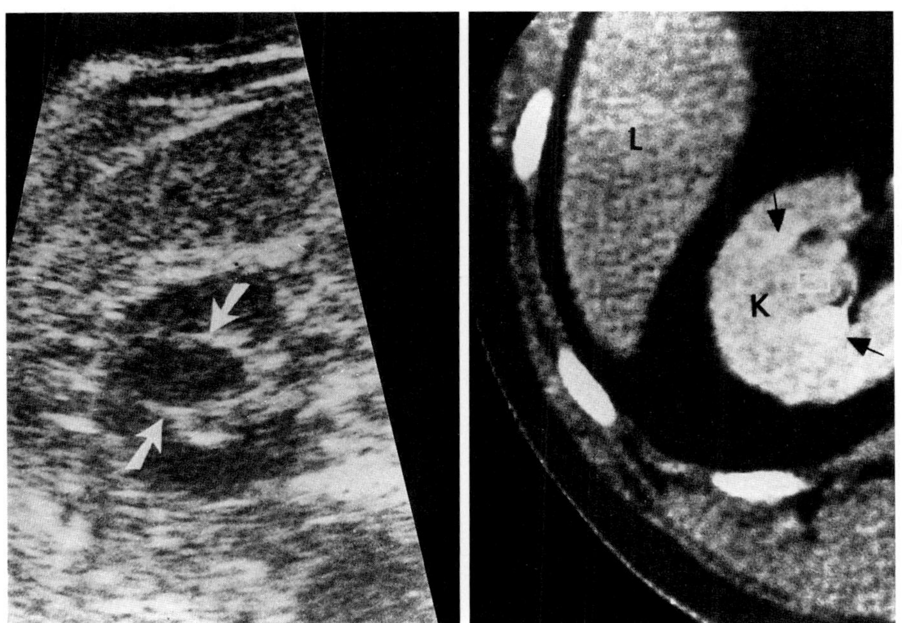

Fig. 19. Case 8. Prominent column of Bertin (*arrows*) on **a** an ultrasonogram and **b** a CT scan. *K*, kidney; *L*, liver

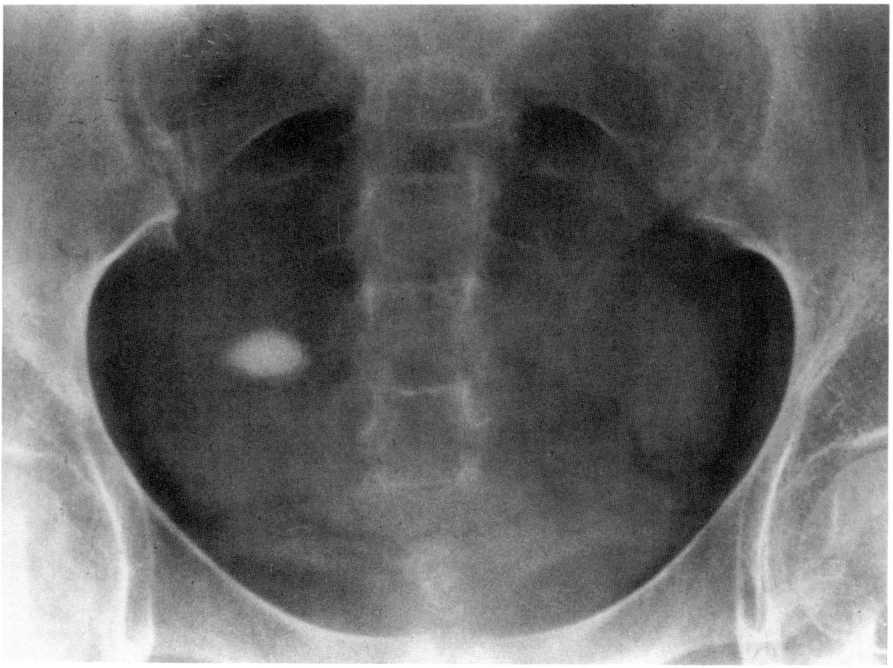

Fig. 20. Case 9. Radiographic appearance in a woman presenting with pain in the hypogastrium. An oval density is present on the right side of the soft tissues of the pelvis, suggesting the presence of a right ureteral calculus or an appendicolith. A urogram was ordered

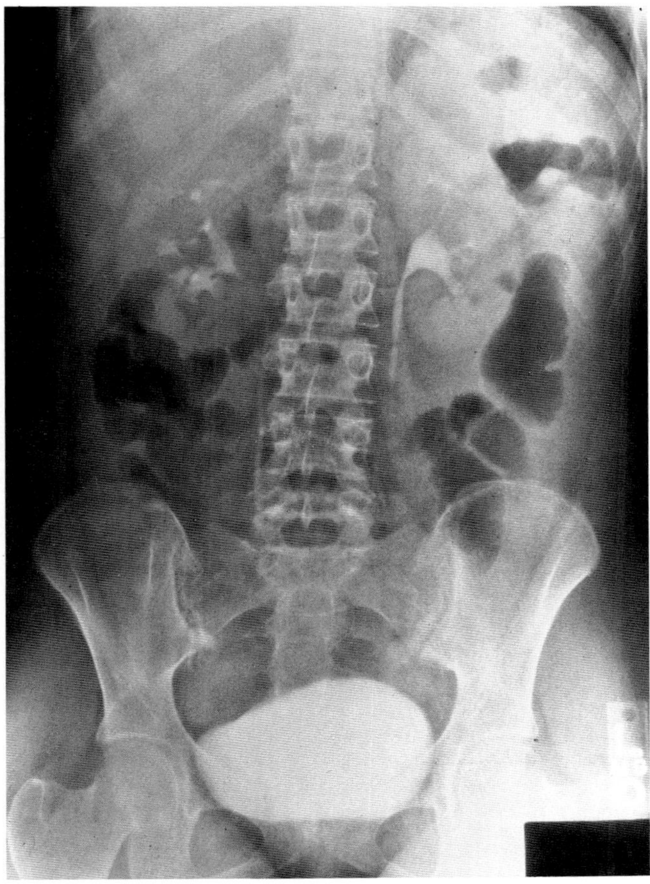

Fig. 21. Case 9. Excretory urogram. Note in this view the presence of the density projected at the lower portion of the right sacroiliac joint

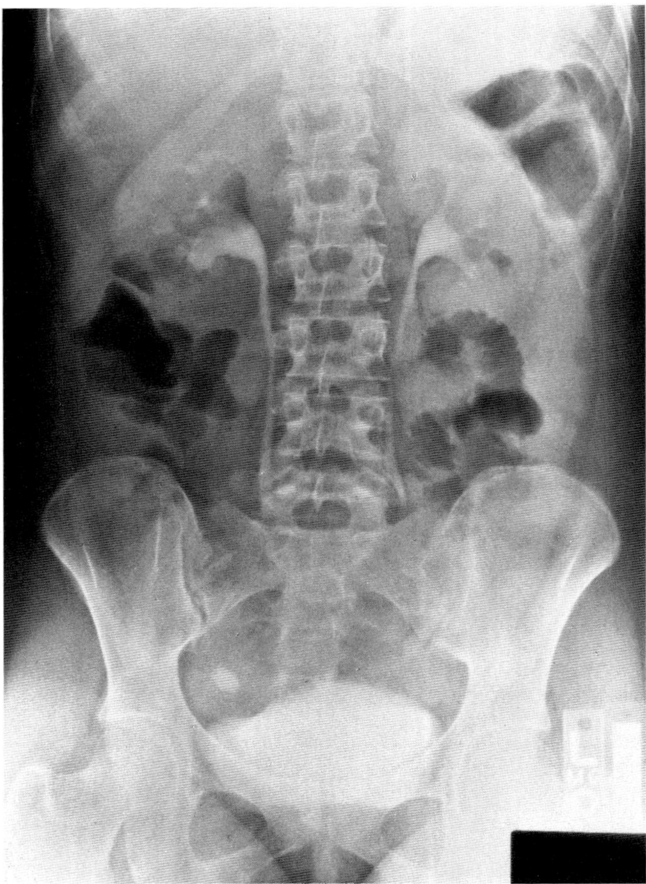

Fig. 22. Case 9. Another excretory urogram obtained during the same procedure as Fig. 21. Note that the density is now located below the right sacroiliac joint

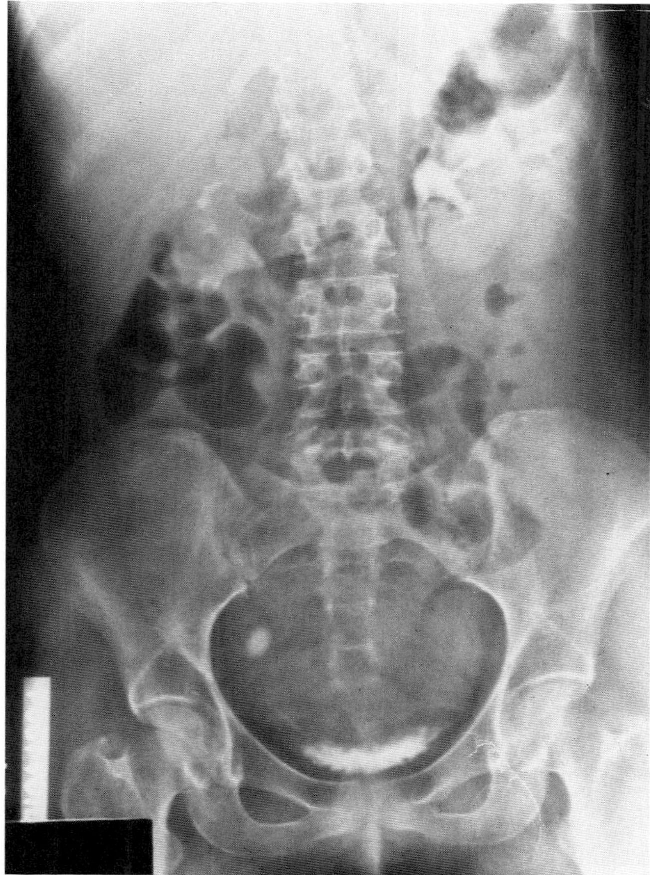

Fig. 23. Case 9. Postevacuation film. Note again the density outside the ureter. The density has changed in position and in orientation. A few hours later the density was not present

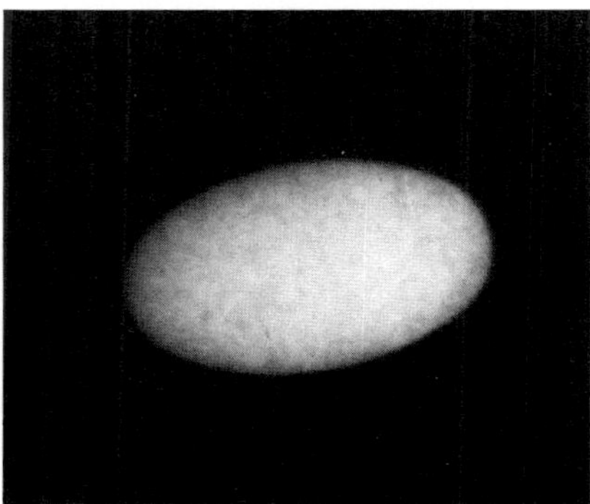

Fig. 24. Case 9. Radiograph of an iron pill taken by the patient

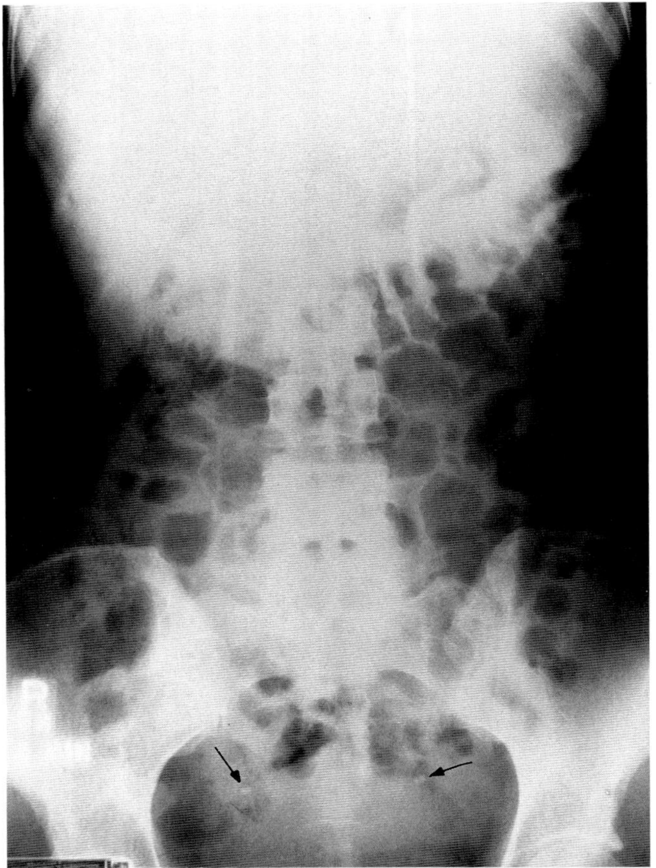

Fig. 25. Case 10. Bilateral densities in the soft tissues of the pelvis in a women who had tubal ligation. Note the characteristic symmetrical morphology of the metallic devices (*arrows*)

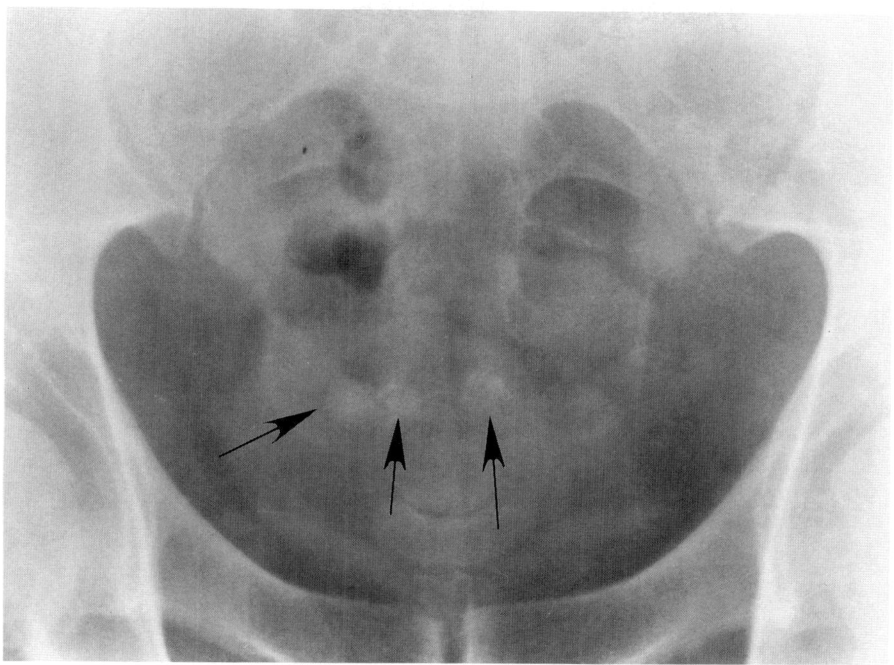

Fig. 26. Case 11. Three densities are evident in the central portion of the pelvis. *Vertical arrows* indicate sacral cornua, the *oblique arrow* the calculus

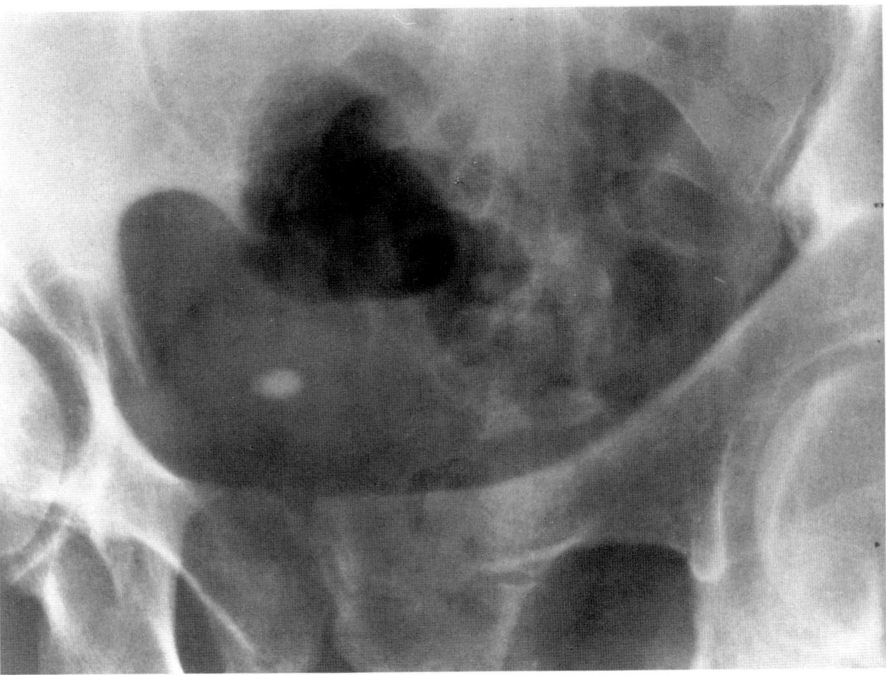

Fig. 27. Case 11. Right posterior oblique projection. One of the densities represents a stone in the bladder. The other two densities, which have a symmetrical distribution, represent the sacral cornua. When the sacral cornua are calcified, they can simulate stones

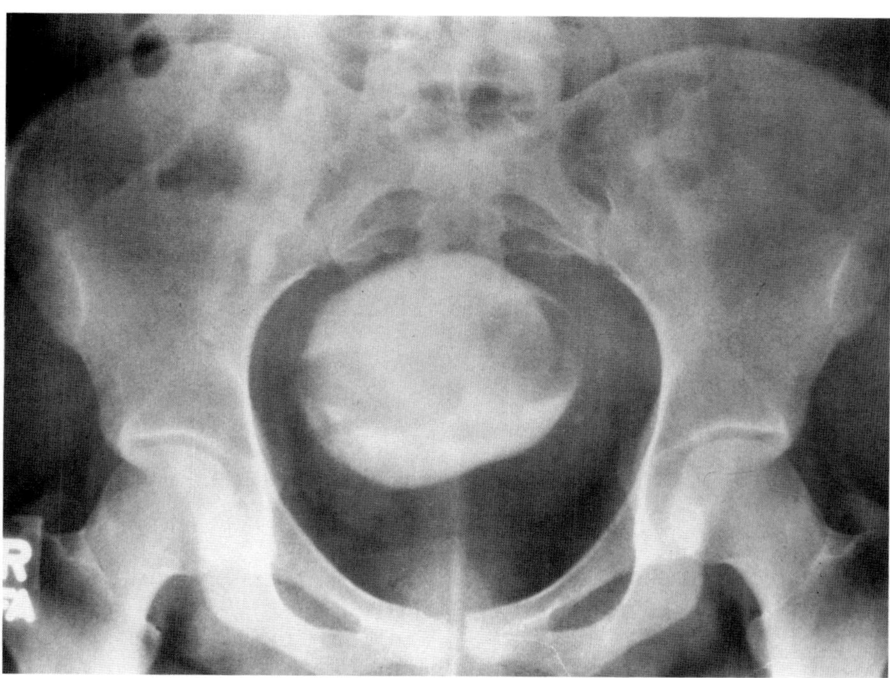

Fig. 28. Case 12. Amniogram. Without a clinical history, the erroneous diagnosis of filling defects in a cystogram could be made. This is a normal amniogram in a patient with a history of anencephaly in previous babies

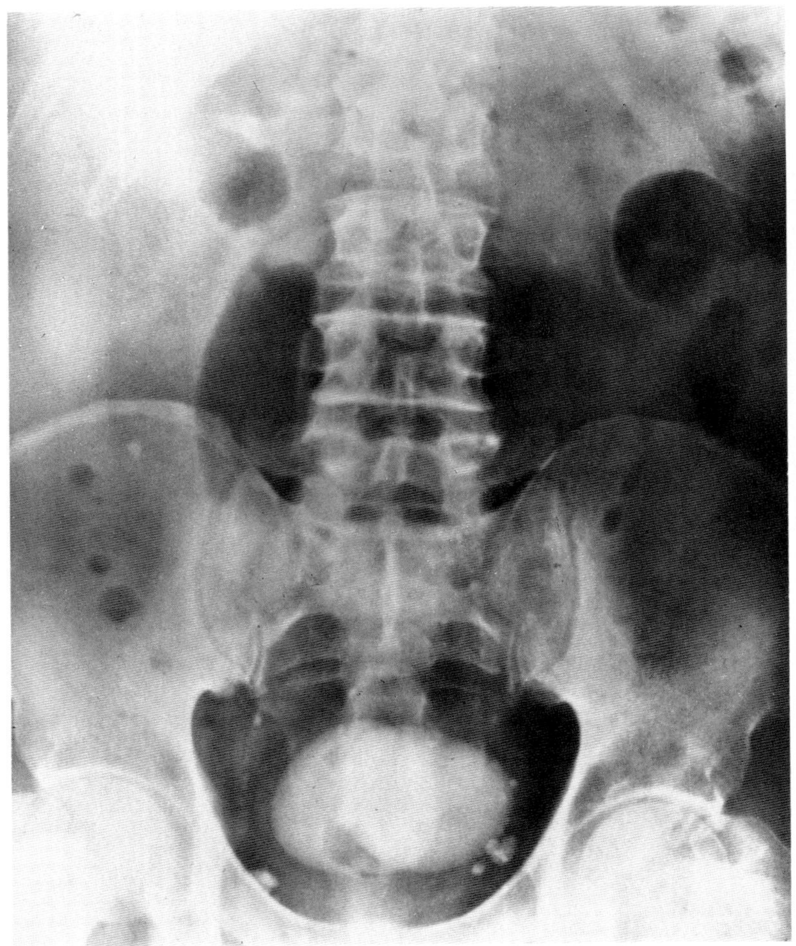

Fig. 29. Case 13. Bladder calculus simulating a cystogram. Clinical information is always very important in avoiding such confusion

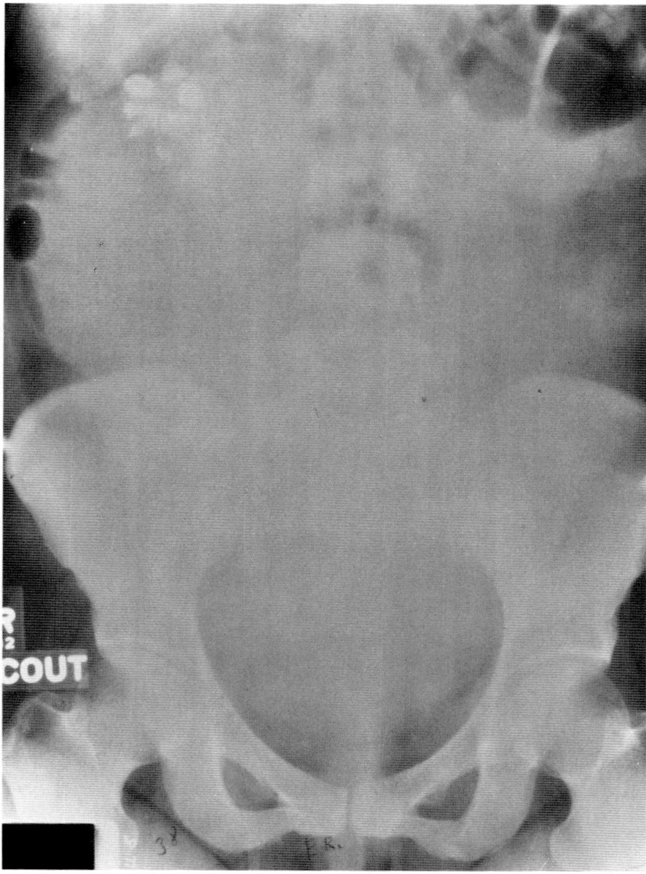

Fig. 30. Case 14. Scout film showing a huge mass with irregular calcification of the right upper quadrant. The diagnosis was massive hydronephrosis and a staghorn calculus

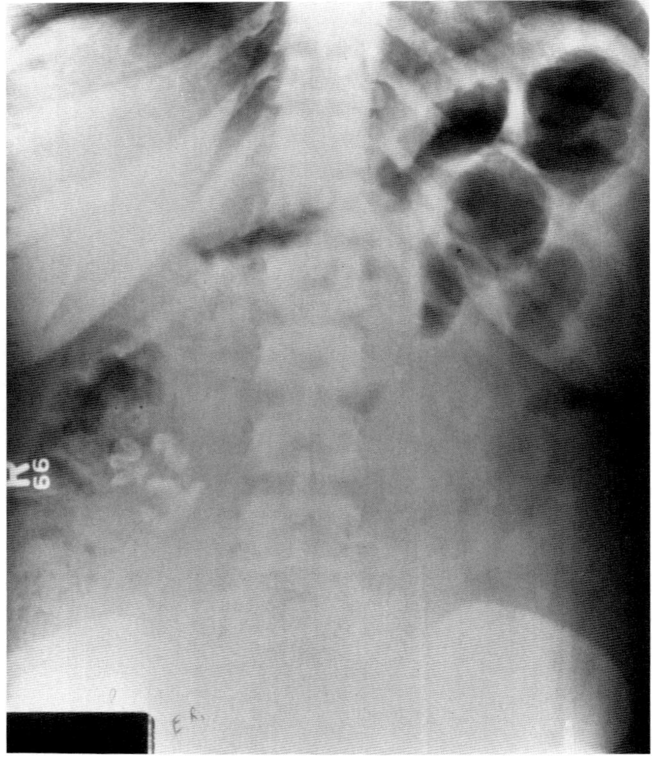

Fig. 31. Case 14. Another scout film shows that the calcifications have the appearance of teeth and bone

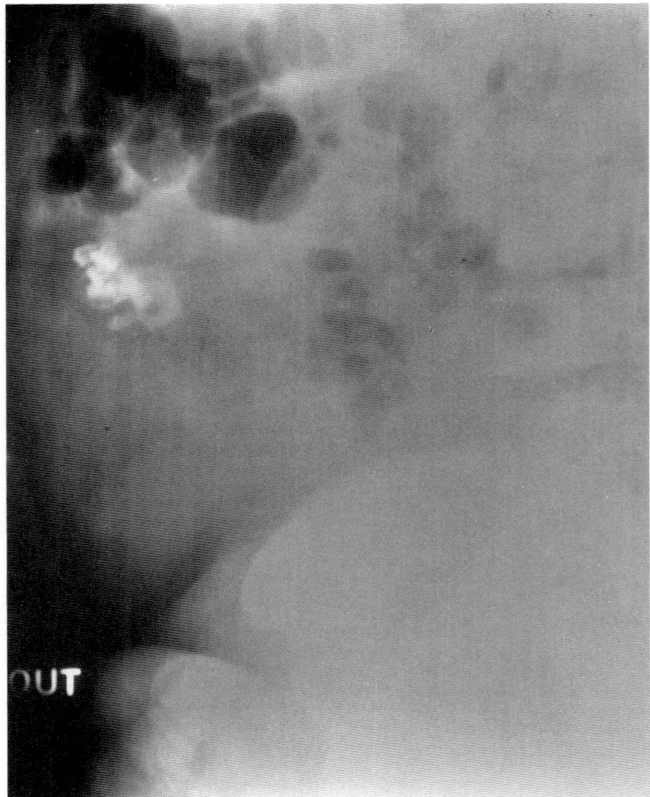

Fig. 32. Case 14. Lateral view showing the anterior location of the calcification, which is seen within a mass. The position of the mass suggests that it is not related to the kidney

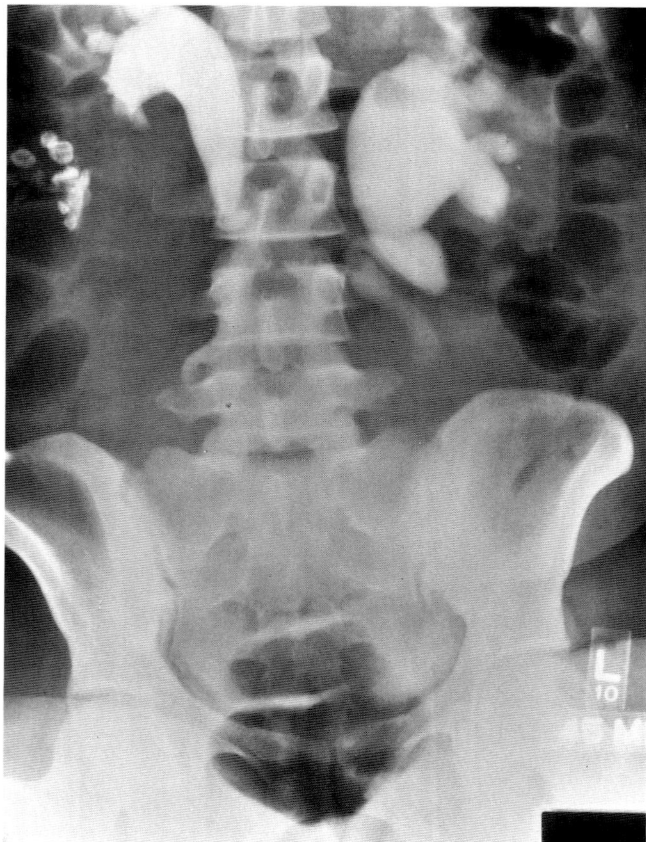

Fig. 33. Case 14. Excretory urogram showing compression of the urinary bladder, bilateral hydronephrosis, and a large mass lateral to the right ureter. At surgery, this proved to be an enlarged uterus with fibromyomas which had displaced superiorly a dermoid of the right ovary

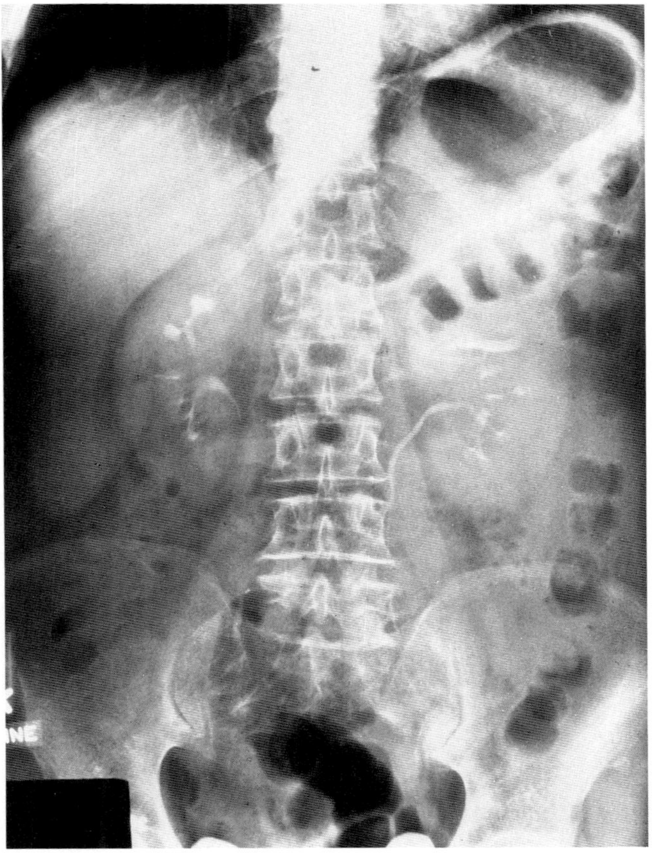

Fig. 34. Case 15. Excretory urogram. The upper pole of the left kidney shows flattening of the left upper calyx and concavity of the superior portion of the left kidney

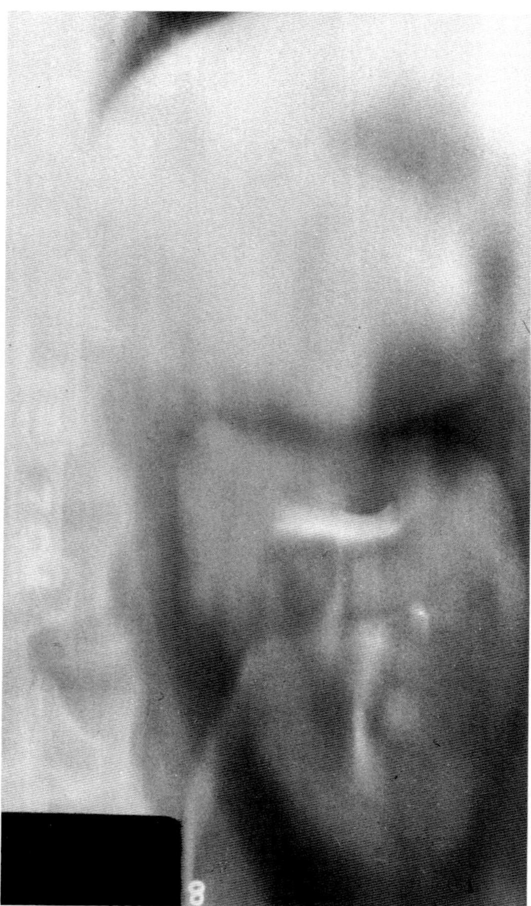

Fig. 35. Case 15. Tomogram revealing a mass above the left kidney. The mass is separate from the upper pole, which appears with a superior concavity. There is flattening of the left upper calyx

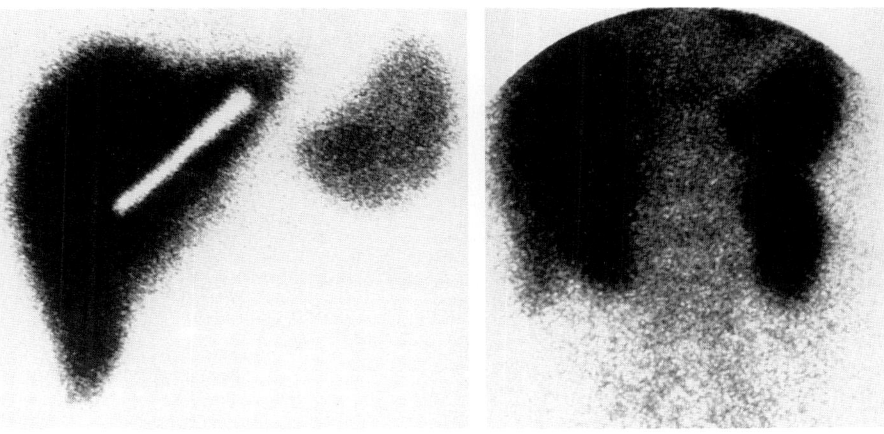

36 37

Fig. 36. Case 15. Liver-spleen scan showing rotated spleen. The lower portion of the spleen is convex, accounting for the topography of the mass observed on the urogram

Fig. 37. Case 15. Liver-spleen scan and renal scan. Superimposition of the two organs confirms the presence of a malrotated spleen which indented the superior pole of the left kidney

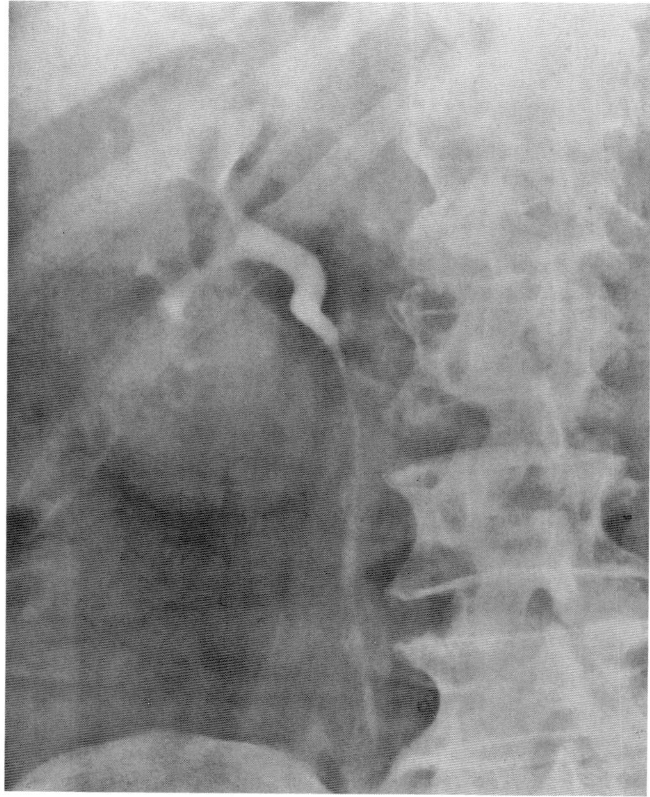

Fig. 38. Case 16. Excretory urogram of the right kidney. Note a mass effect in the topography of the lower portion of the right kidney

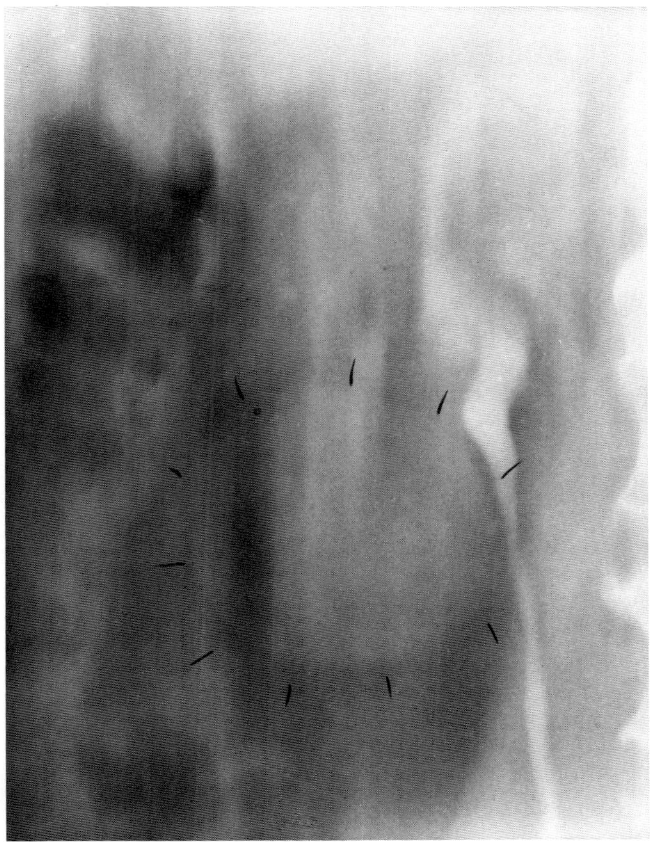

Fig. 39. Case 16. Nephrotomogram. A rounded density appears in the topography of the lower pole of the right kidney. Note that it has a superior margin

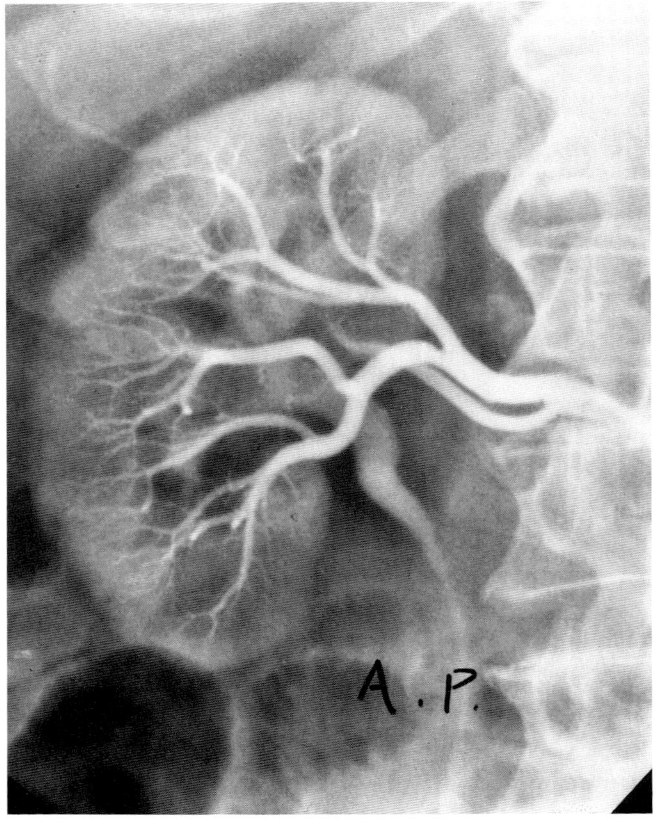

Fig. 40. Case 16. Selective right renal arteriogram, frontal projection. The mass is no longer seen. This was a perfectly normal study

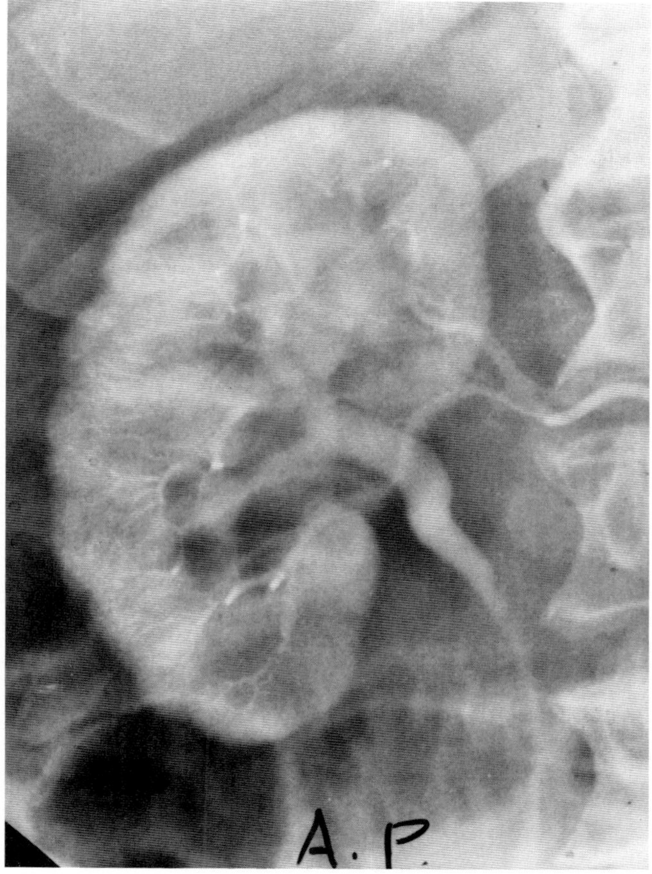

Fig. 41. Case 16. Late phase of the selective renal arteriogram showing no evidence of a mass

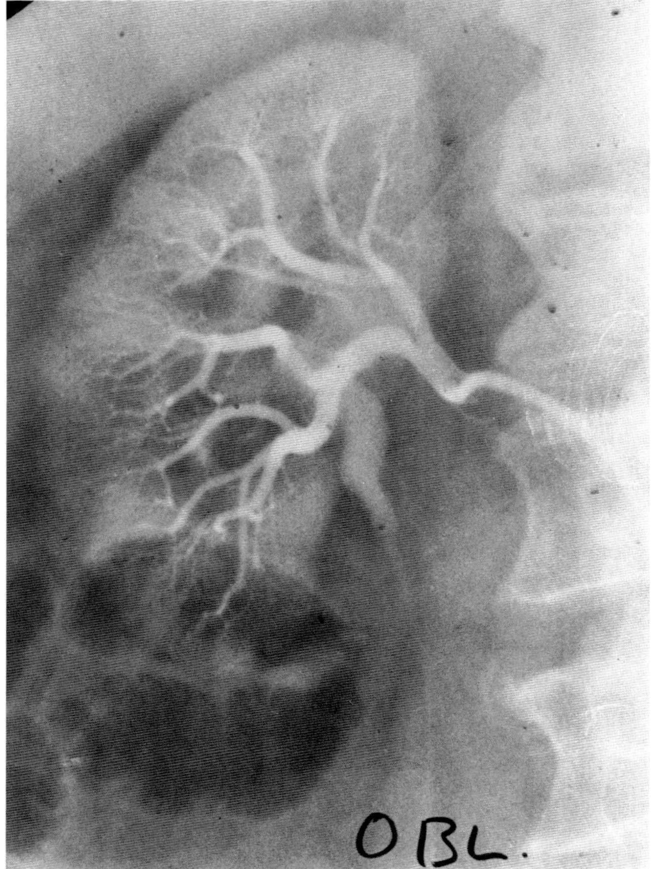

Fig. 42. Case 16. Right posterior oblique view of a selective right renal arteriogram. There is no evidence of a mass

In retrospect, films should have been obtained with the patient prone or upright. By changing the position of the patient, fluid in the bowel would have shifted and the "tumor" would have disappeared

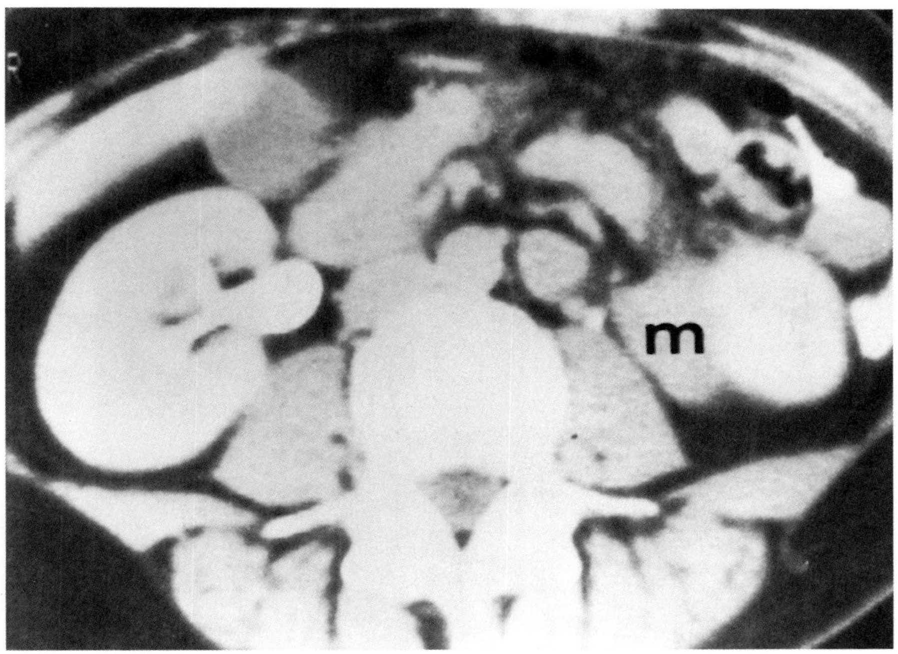

Fig. 43. Case 17. CT of the retroperitoneum revealing a mass (*m*) medial to the left kidney

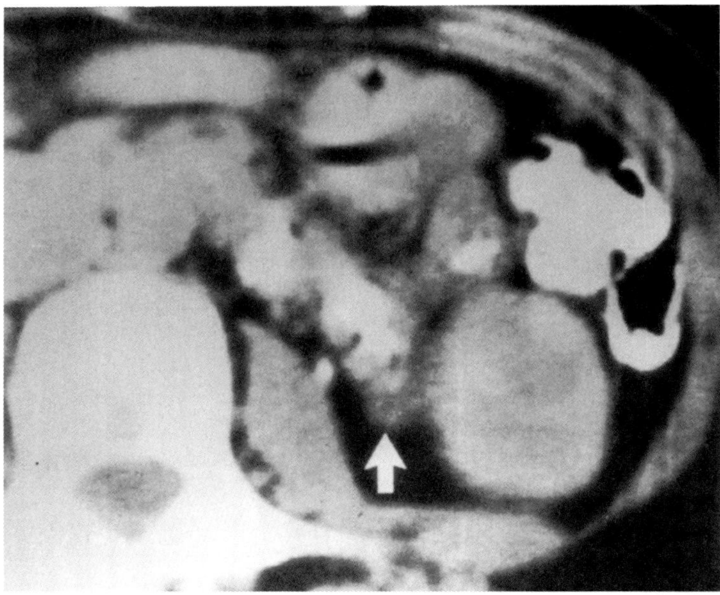

Fig. 44. Case 17. Appearance following administration of an oral contrast agent. The mass has opacified and is seen to correspond to a bowel loop (*arrow*)

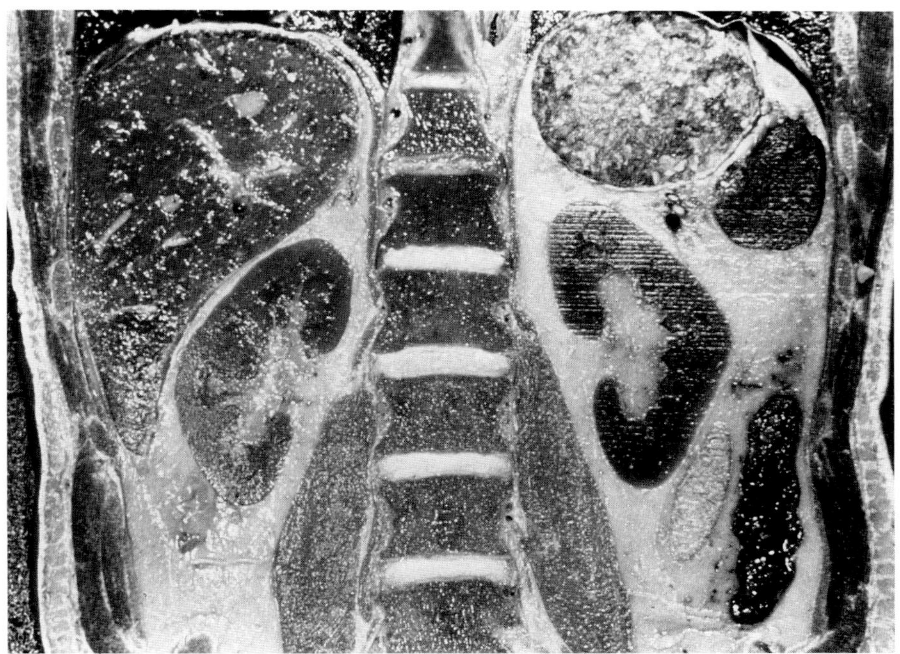

Fig. 45. Coronal anatomic section at the level of the kidneys. Note the anatomical contiguity of the hila with the perirenal fat

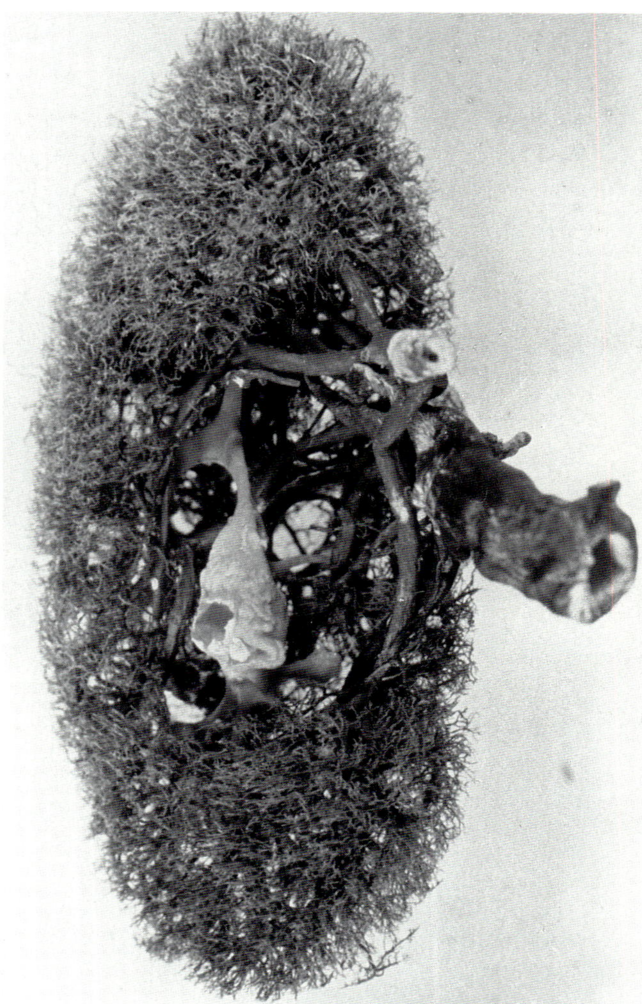

Fig. 46. Cast corrosion preparation of a normal left kidney, medial view. Note separation of the light-colored renal pelvis from the surrounding arteries and veins. The space between the pelvocalyceal system and the vessels is occupied by fat. Fat allows distensibility of the renal pelvis in individuals with an intrarenal pelvis. Fat is of less significance when a person has an extrarenal pelvis. Excessive fat in the renal sinus in a patient with an extrarenal pelvis should make one suspect a pathological condition, although it can represent an anatomical variant

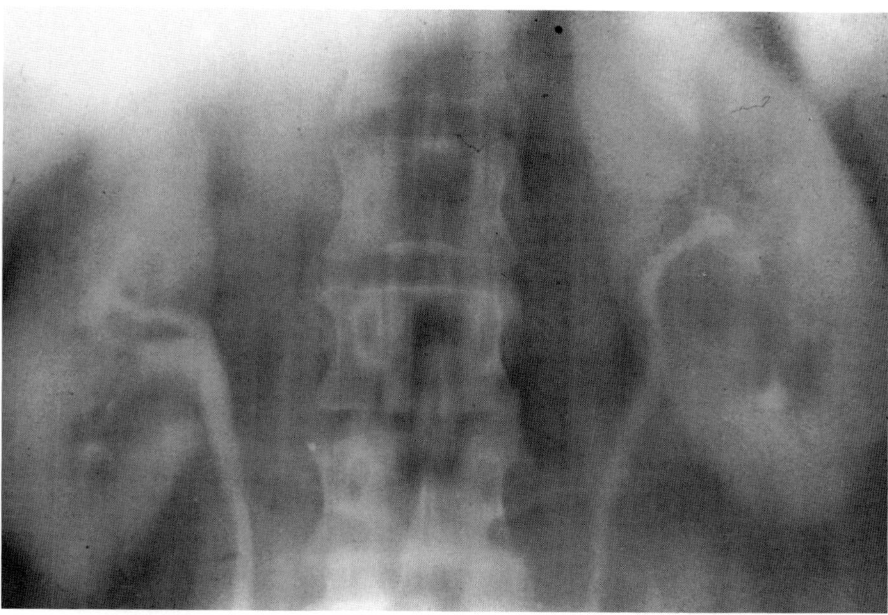

Fig. 47. Nephrotomogram showing normal renal hili. Note radiolucency in the central medial portion of the kidneys around the renal pelvis and infundibuli. This represents the fat in the renal sinus

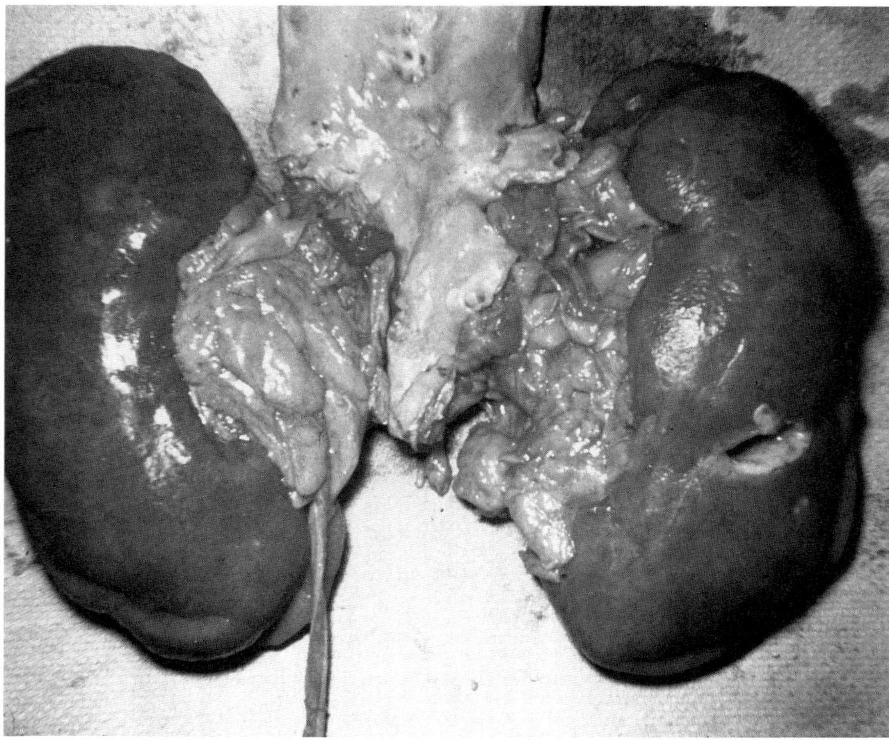

Fig. 48. Specimen showing excessive fat in the renal hilus in a patient with papillary necrosis

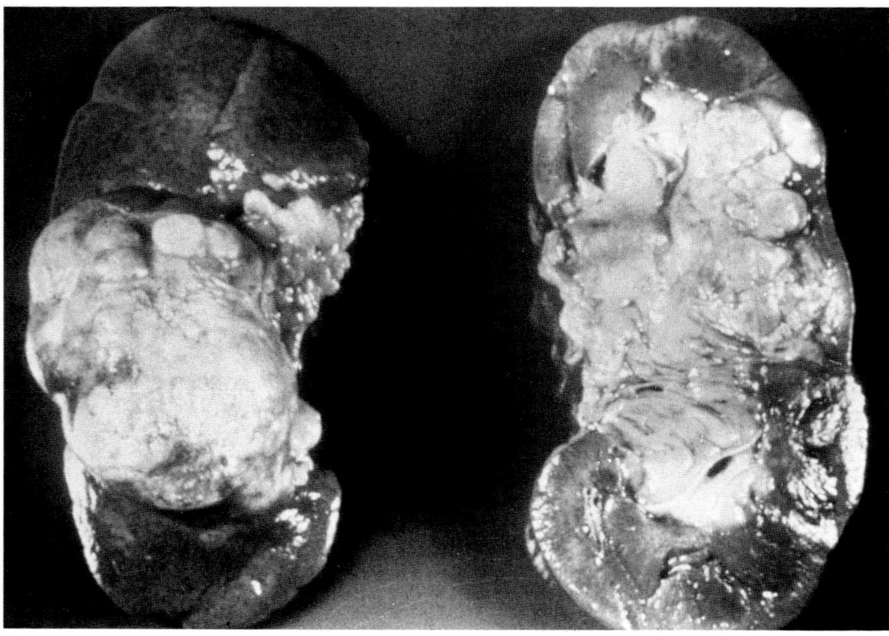

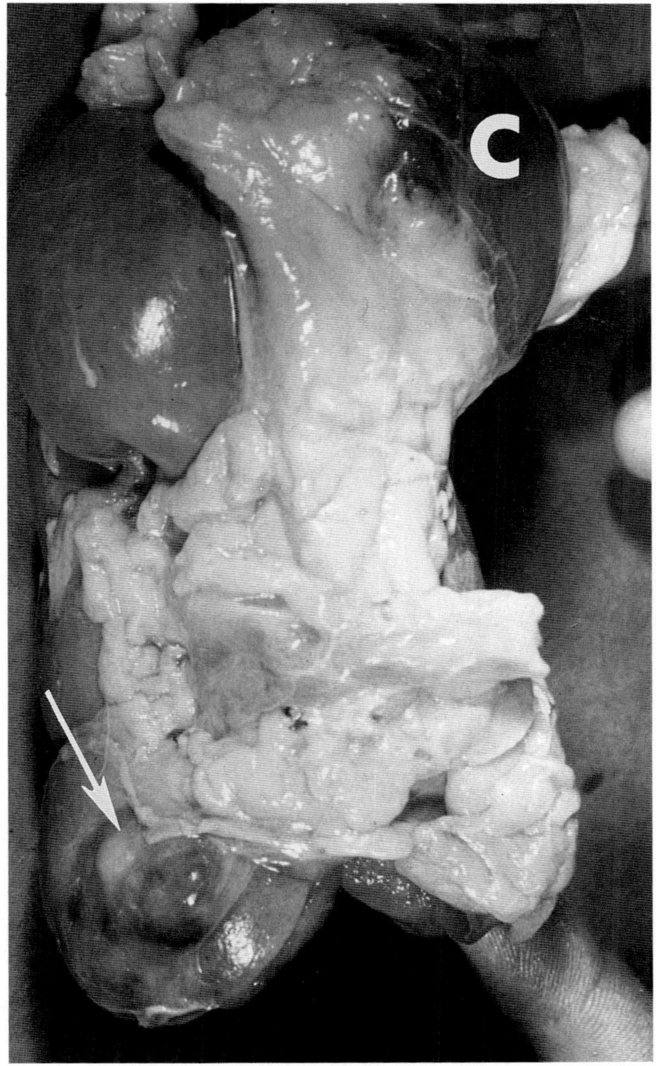

Fig. 49. Specimen from a patient with a carcinoma in the lower pole of the left kidney (*arrow*) and a cyst (*C*) in the upper pole of the same kidney. Note excessive fat in the medial aspect of the left kidney

◄

Fig. 50. Excessive fat in the mid portion of the left kidney due to angiomyolipoma

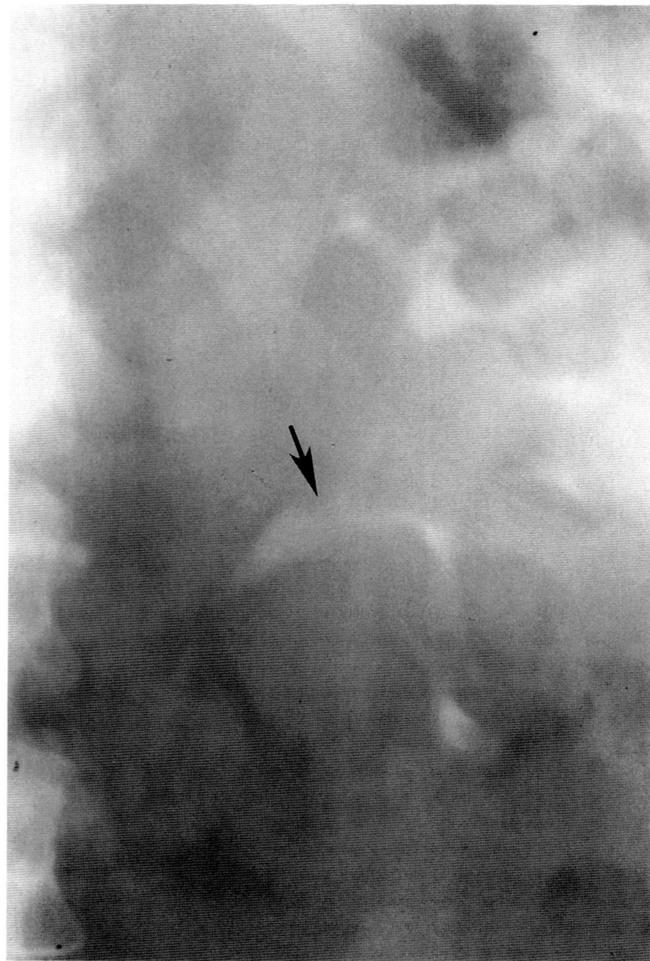

Fig. 51. Case 18. Excretory urogram from an 18-year-old woman who had lost weight on the basis of a rigid diet. She presented with flank pain. A filling defect is seen in the upper portion of the left renal pelvis (*arrow*), simulating a stone, a clot, or a tumor. Note the absence of fat in the renal sinus

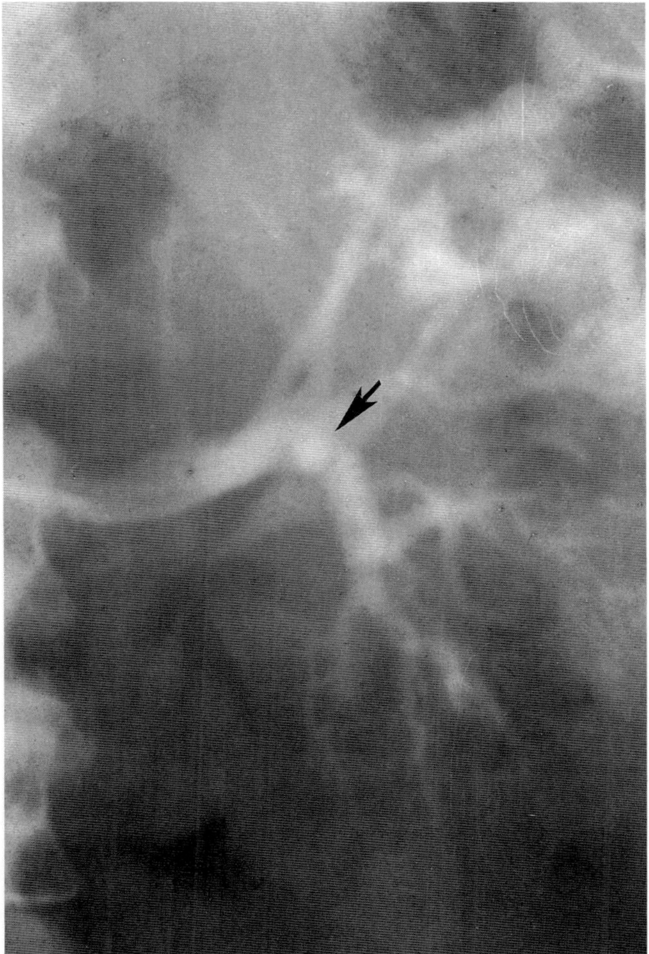

Fig. 52. Case 18. Selective left renal arteriogram. Note a branch of the dorsal renal artery (*arrow*) indenting the superior portion of the left renal pelvis. The absence of fat caused the proximity of vessels to the pelvocalyceal system. Whenever indentation affects the infundibuli or renal pelvis in a patient with no fat in the sinus, one should entertain the diagnosis of a vascular impression, which may be the result of absence of fat. No tumor was found in this patient

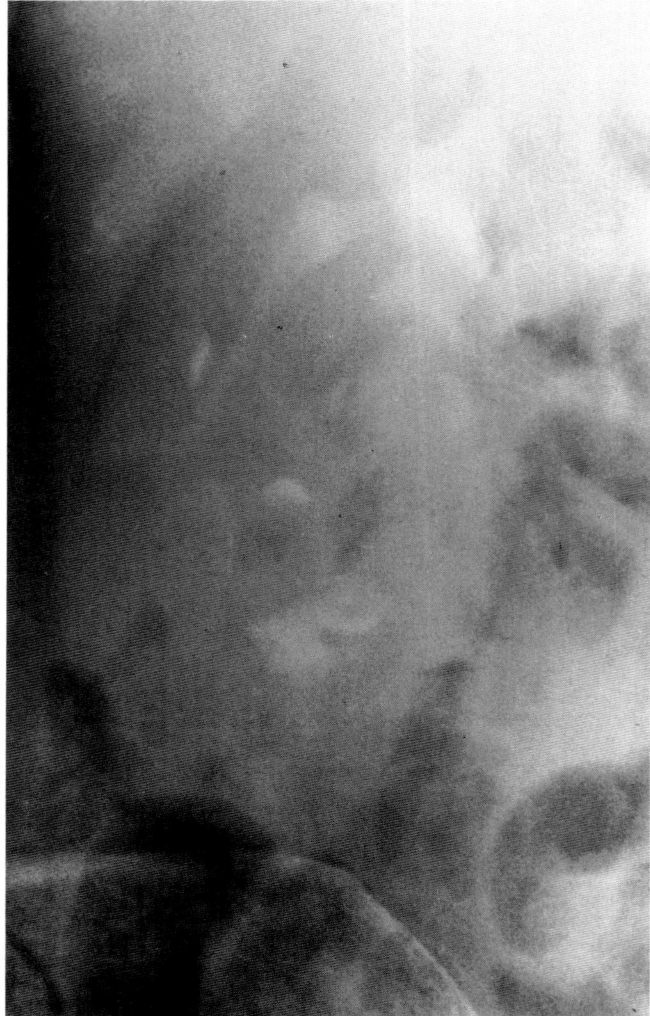

Fig. 53. Case 19. Excretory urogram showing a mass effect in the central portion of the right kidney with compression of the renal pelvis and mild internal hydronephrosis. The mass was thought to represent a neoplasm and was secondary to a renal arteriovenous fistula. The patient presented with cardiomegaly, congestive heart failure, and hematuria. He gave a history of being stabbed in the flank 2 years previously

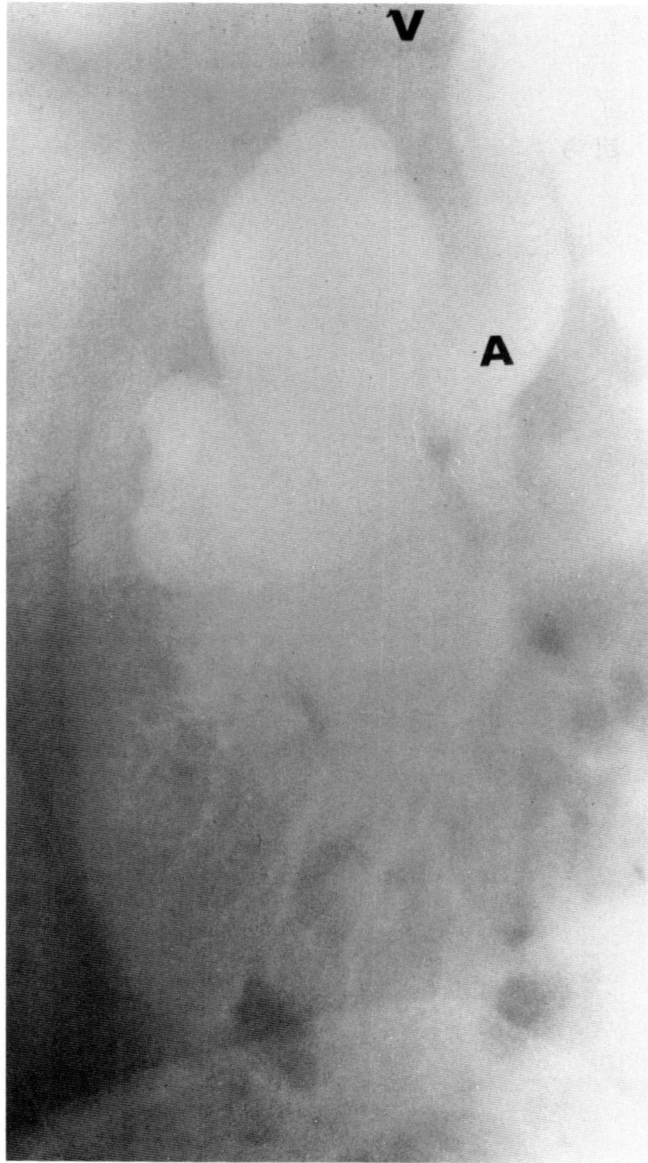

Fig. 54. Case 19. Selective right renal arteriogram showing the huge right renal artery (*A*), the collection of contrast medium at the level of the arteriovenous communication, and a large draining vein (*V*)

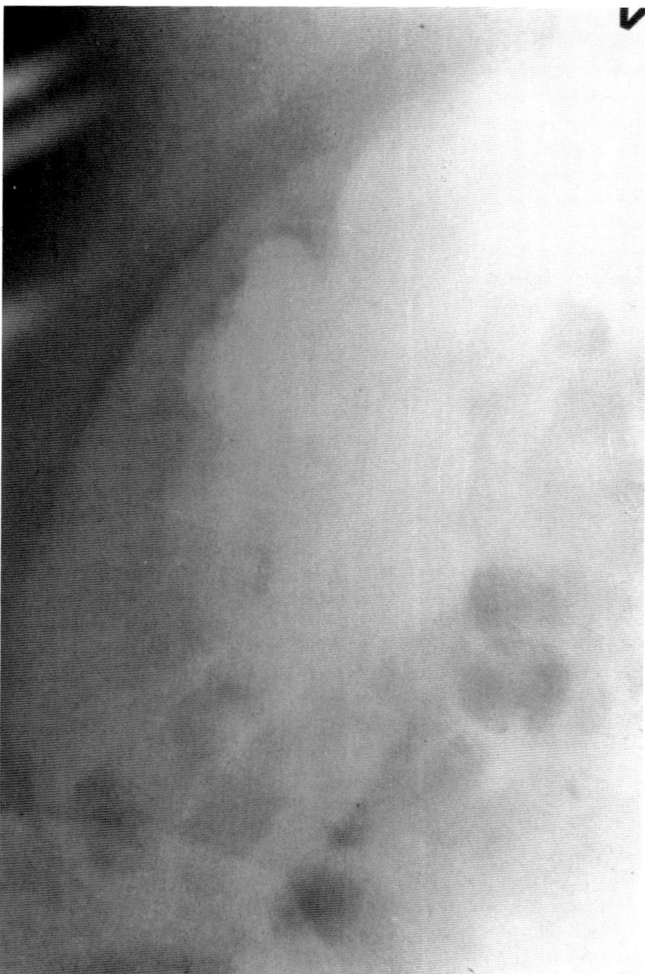

Fig. 55. Case 19. Venous phase of a selective right renal arteriogram. Note the arteriovenous fistula and the large draining vein (*V*). An astute surgical resident auscultated the right flank and made the diagnosis of an arteriovenous fistula based on clinical information and physical findings. In some instances the stethoscope exceeds in value radiographic methods

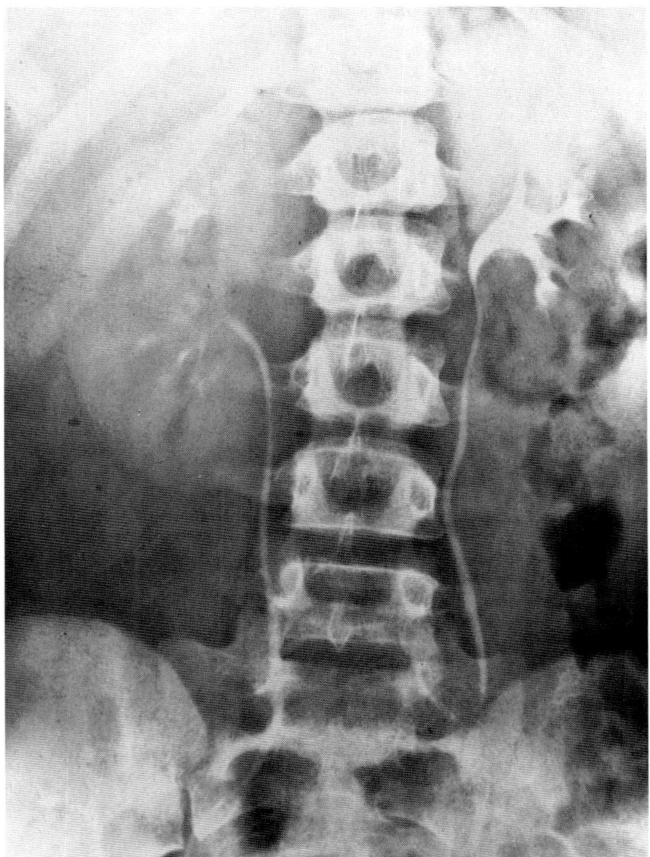

Fig. 56. Case 20. Excretory urogram of a child who fell from a ladder, hitting his right flank. He presented with hematuria. The urogram shows decreased opacification of the right pelvocalyceal system. The right kidney is enlarged and a large defect is noted in its central portion. An arteriogram was ordered

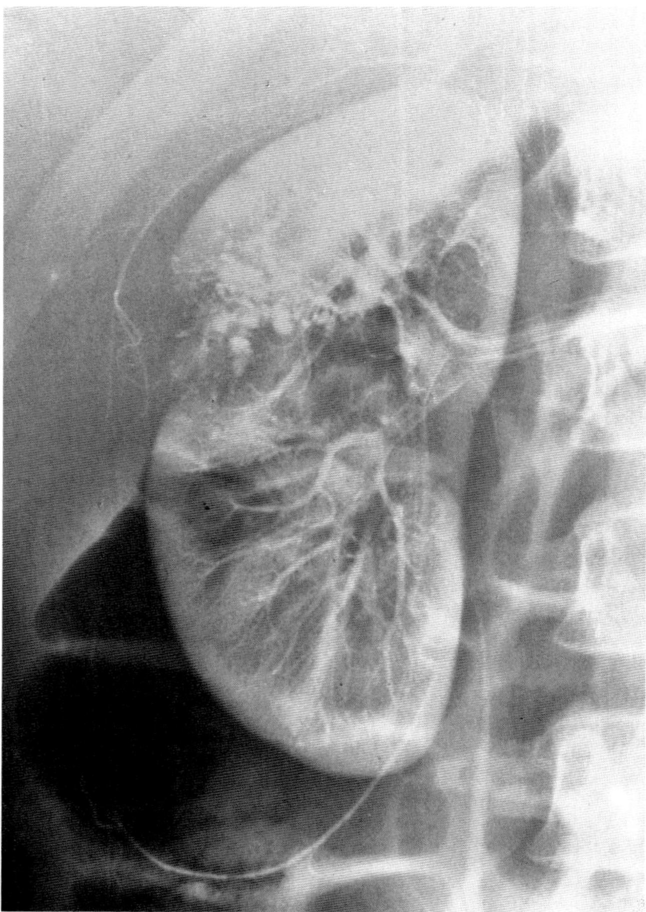

Fig. 57. Case 20. Selective right renal arteriogram, late arterial phase. Note small aneurysms, a defect in the outer portion of the right kidney, and lateral displacement of the capsular artery suggesting the presence of a perirenal hematoma. The urologist entertained the possibility of a Wilms' tumor or an angiomyolipoma and decided to "explore" the patient

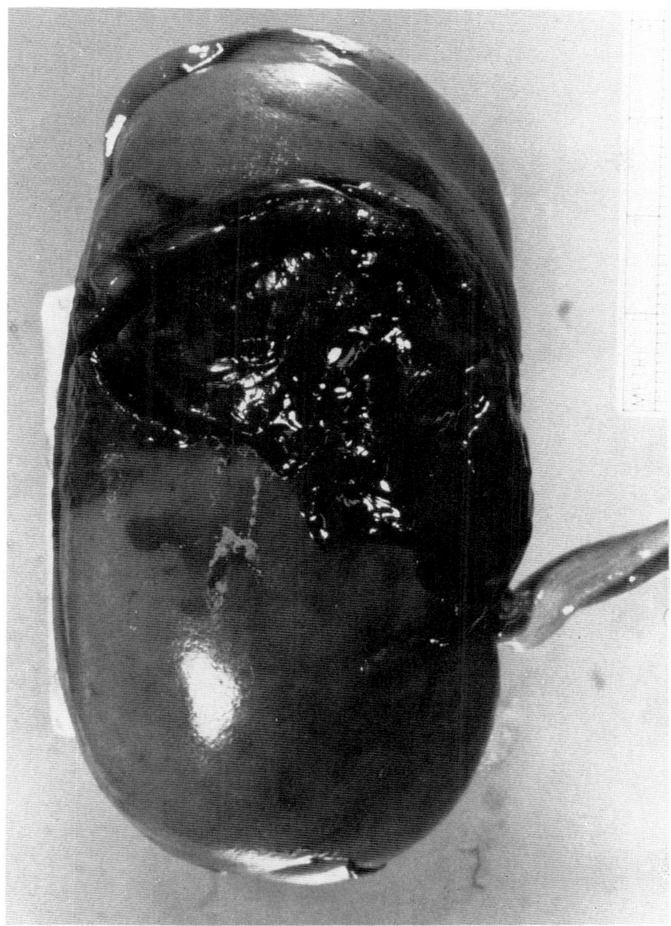

Fig. 58. Case 20. Photograph of the right kidney at surgery. Note laceration of the kidney and an area of hemorrhage

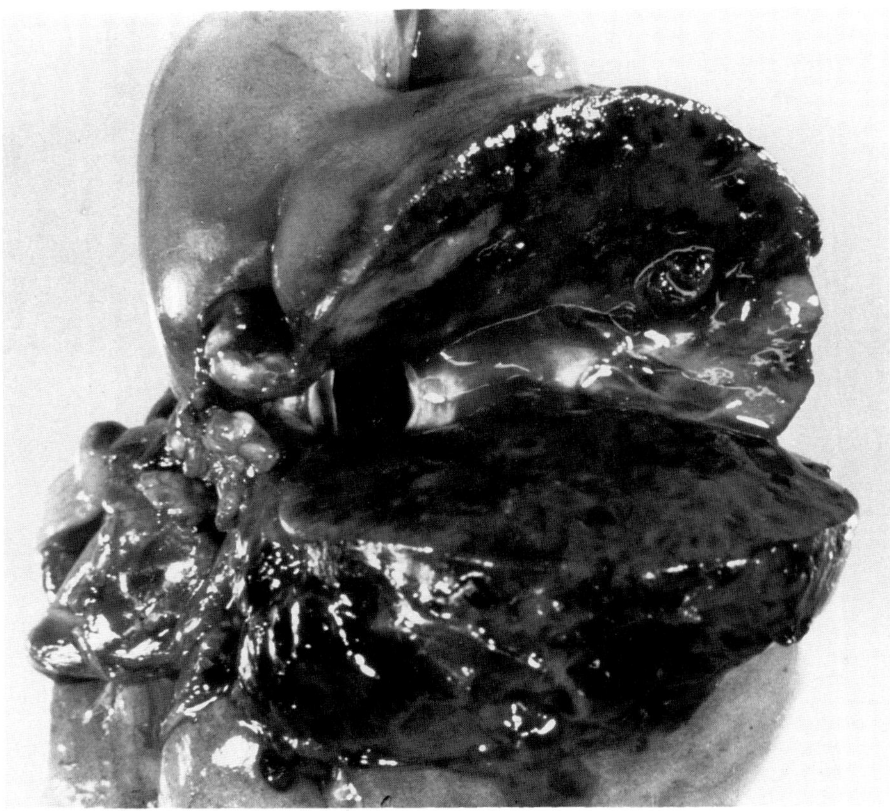

Fig. 59. Case 20. Close-up of sectioned right kidney. Note an area of hemorrhage. No tumor was found

Contusion of solid organs can lead to small collections of contrast material when arteriography is performed. Such collections can simulate aneurysms found in polyarteritis nodosa, renal angiomyolipomas, neoplasms, and metastatic myxomas. Whenever trauma has occurred, a mass effect in a solid organ should be considered to be a hematoma and conservative management is usually indicated. Repeat examination and, particularly, the use of noninvasive modalities such as ultrasonography, CT, or MRI will show regression of the mass if there is a hematoma. Persistence of the mass may warrant biopsy or surgical exploration.

In my experience, when surgeons talk about exploration, the patient loses one or more organs, or parts thereof!

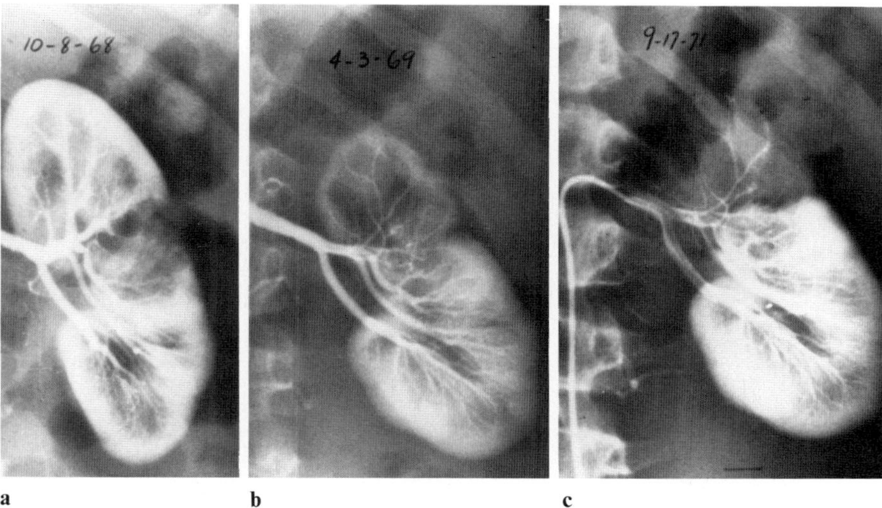

Fig. 60 a–c. Case 21. **a** Selective left renal arteriogram of a patient who had trauma to the left kidney. Note a mass in the central portion of the left kidney and interruption of the renal cortex. This was due to a hematoma. Subsequent radiographs taken **b** 6 months and **c** almost 3 years later show progressive atrophy of the upper third of the left kidney. Indeed, by the time of the latter radiograph there was almost complete disappearance of the upper pole of the left kidney and compensatory hypertrophy of the lower pole. Such a finding is usually the result of decompensated segmental renal vein obstruction, chronic obstructive uropathy, or segmental uropathy

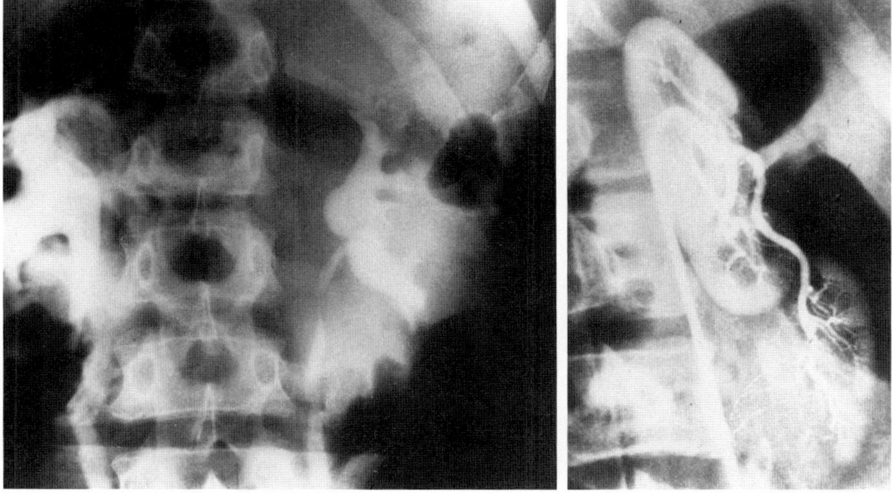

Fig. 61a, b. Case 22. **a** Excretory urogram of a patient with left renal trauma, showing discrete indentation of the medial aspect of the left renal pelvis. **b** Selective left renal arteriography a few days later shows, in the left posterior oblique projection, total disruption of the left kidney, with the lower pole connected to the main kidney by a branch of the left renal artery. A situation like this warrants immediate surgical exploration. Disruption of this vessel can lead to a fatal hemorrhage. Fracture of the left kidney was not suspected clinically, or by urography

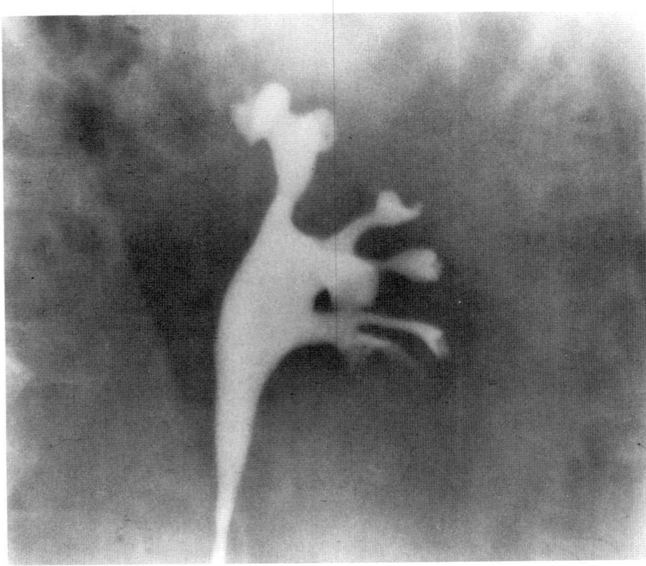

Fig. 62. Case 23. Excretory urogram of a patient who presented with left-sided hematuria. The patient was taking anticoagulants and had suffered a recent heart attack. Note a mass effect in the lower pole of the left kidney with superior displacement of a lower calyx

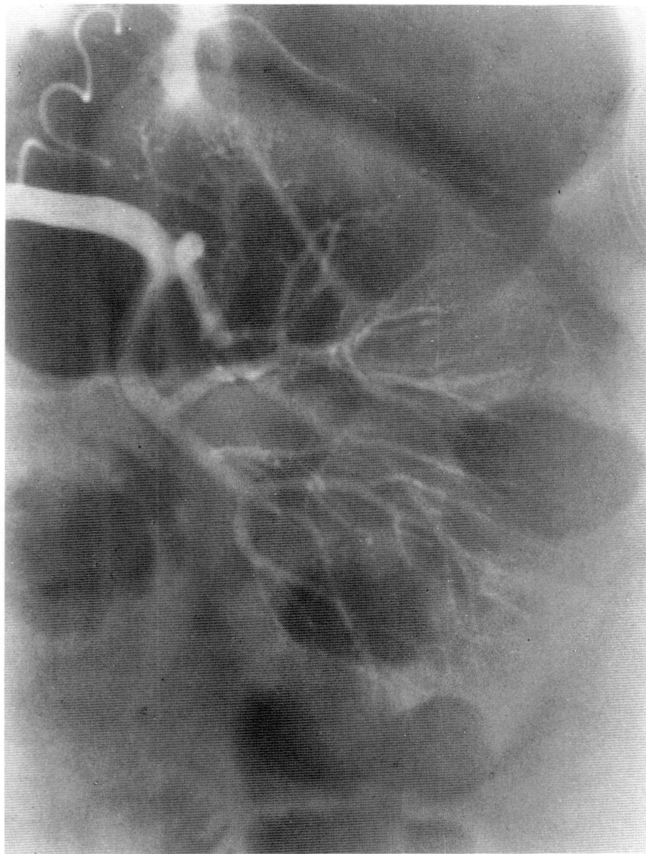

Fig. 63. Case 23. Selective left renal arteriogram. No mass is seen. The intrarenal arteries appear normal radiographically

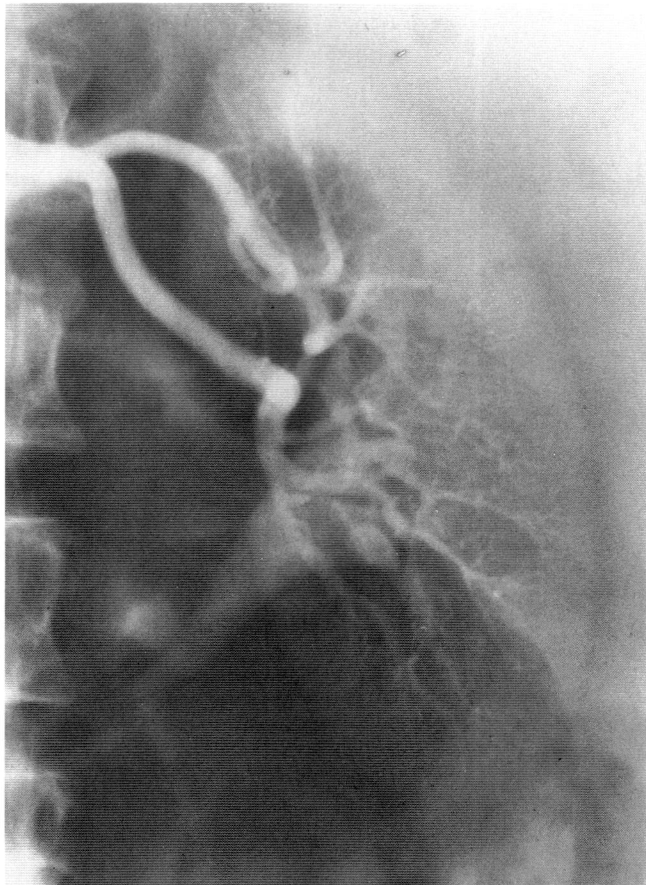

Fig. 64. Case 23. Left posterior oblique study of the left renal arteriogram. No mass is noted, nor is there any evidence of neovascularity. The left kidney was removed

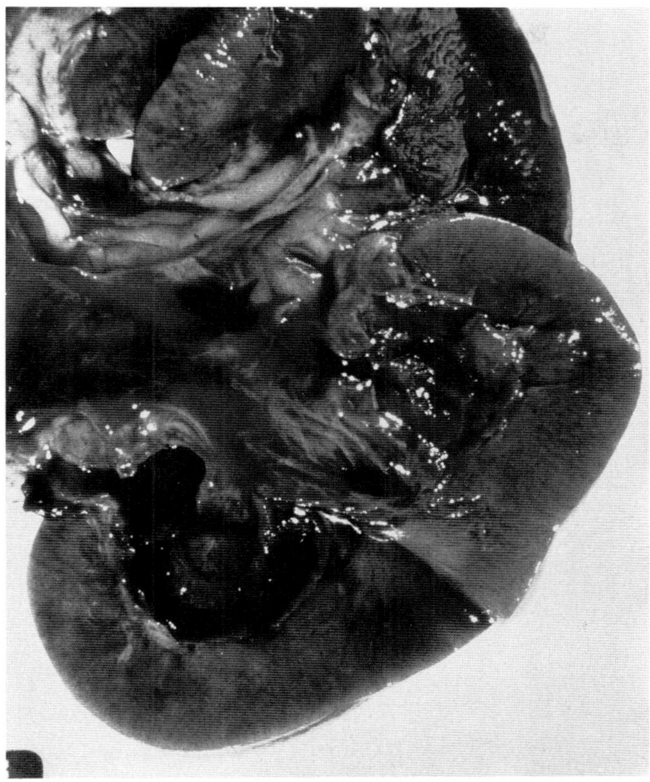

Fig. 65. Case 23. Open specimen of the lower pole of the left kidney. Note an area of hemorrhage in the lower pole of the left kidney. No tumor was found. There was no evidence of infection or of a vascular anomaly. An Antopol-Goldman lesion had been responsible for the original simulation of a renal neoplasm

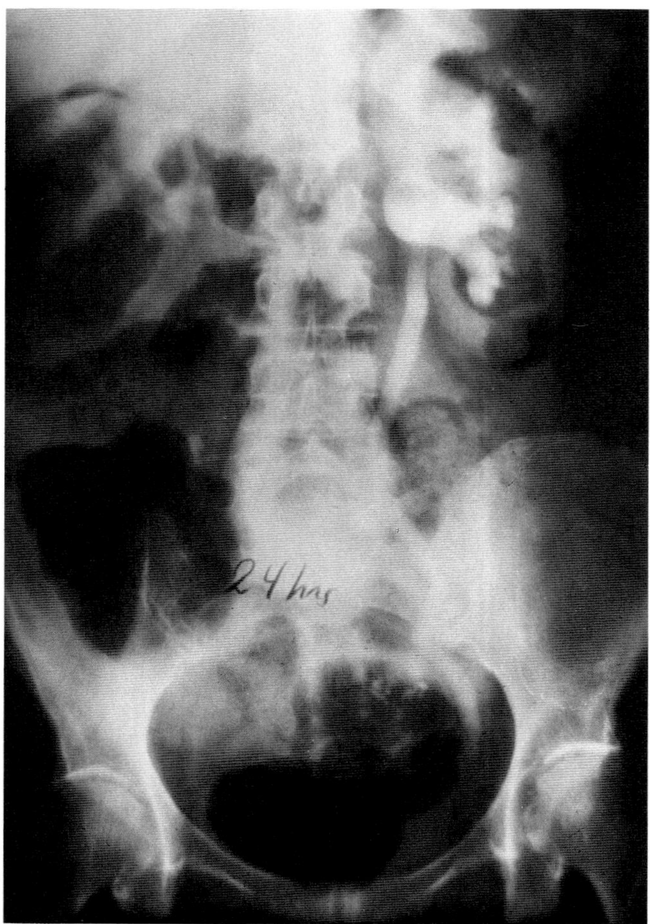

Fig. 66. Case 24. Late phase of an excretory urogram (24 h after the injection of contrast medium) in a patient who presented with left flank pain and hematuria. The patient was also on anticoagulants. Note hydronephrosis of the left kidney and several filling defects in the left renal pelvis and proximal left ureter

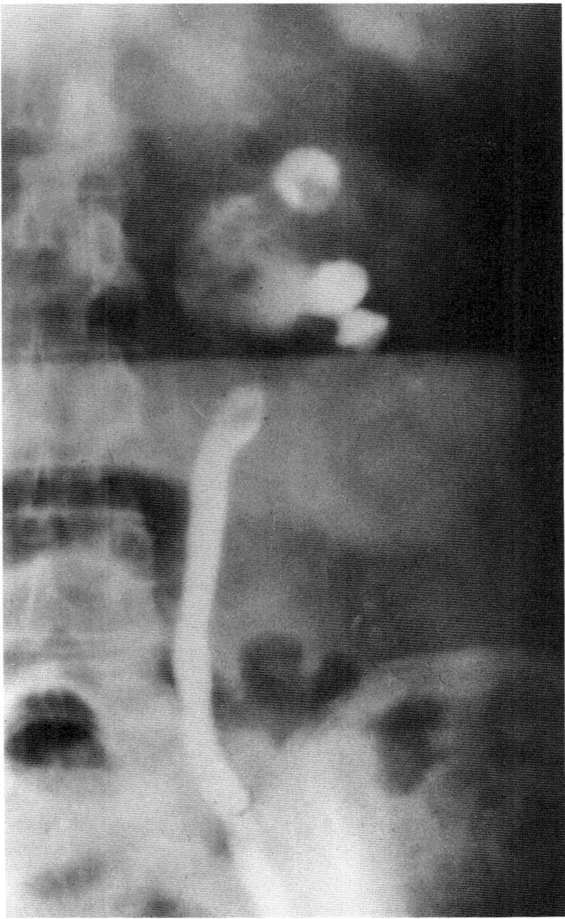

Fig. 67. Case 24. Left retrograde study showing filling defects in the left renal pelvis as well as throughout the left ureter. An arteriogram was ordered

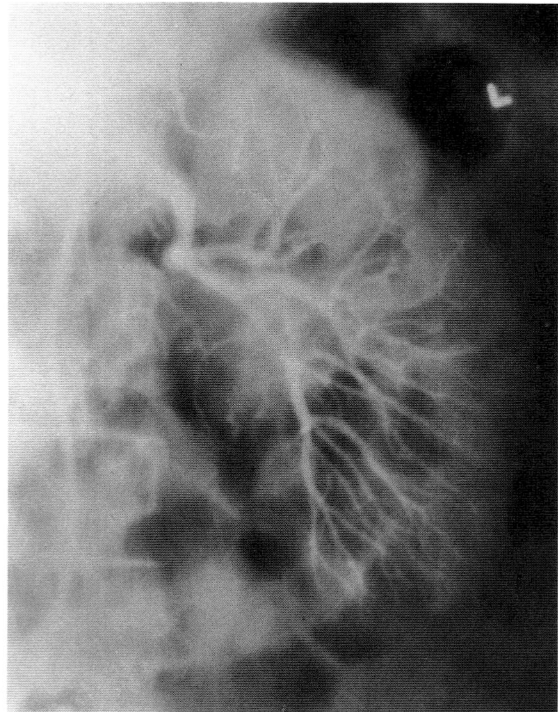

Fig. 68. Case 24. Selective left renal arteriogram, early phase. Note normal findings

Fig. 70. Case 24. Arteriogram following injection of epinephrine. Note uniform constriction of vessels with no evidence of neovascularity. The left kidney was removed

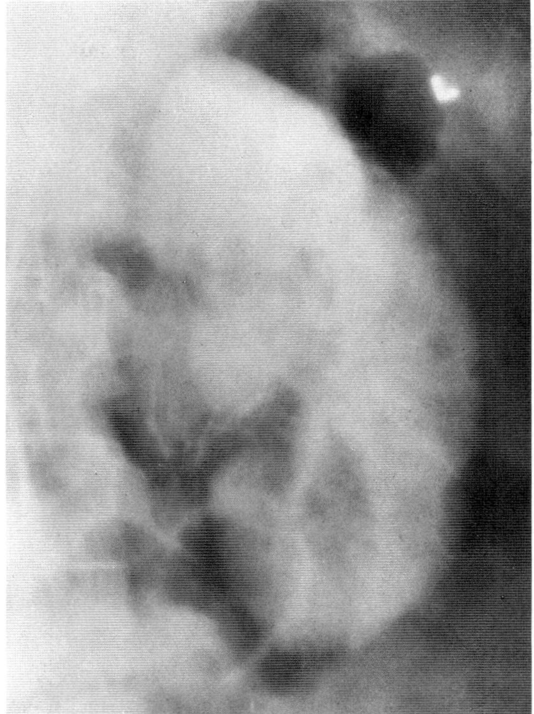

Fig. 69. Case 24. Selective left renal arteriogram, late phase. No abnormalities were noted

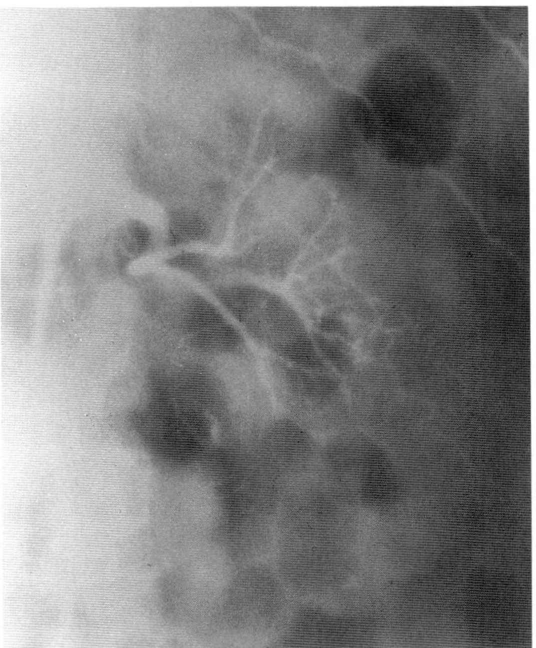

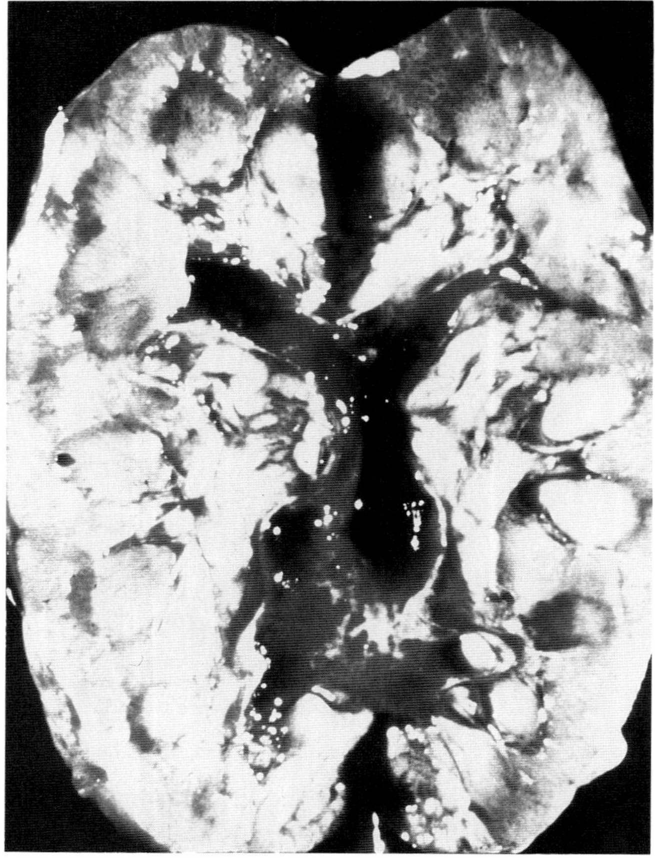

Fig. 71. Case 24. Open left kidney showing clots in the left renal pelvis

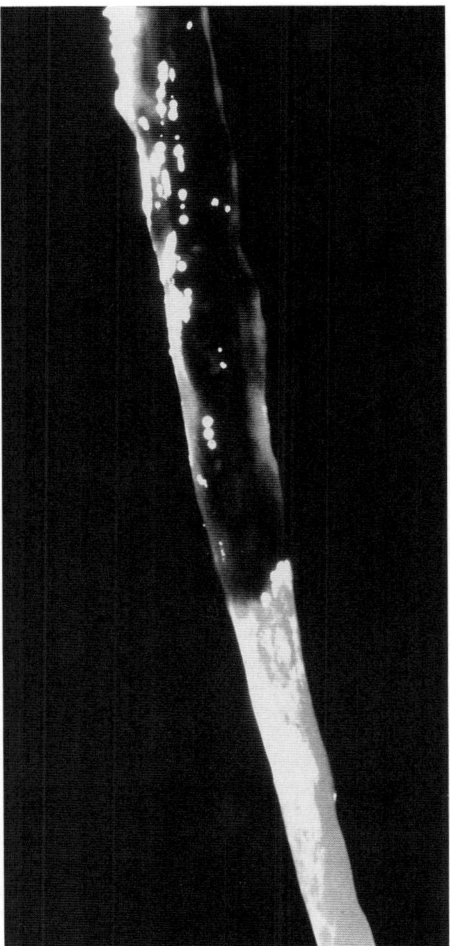

Fig. 72. Case 24. Left ureter open. Note clots in the left ureter. On careful histological sectioning, no tumor was found. A subepithelial hemorrhage was present

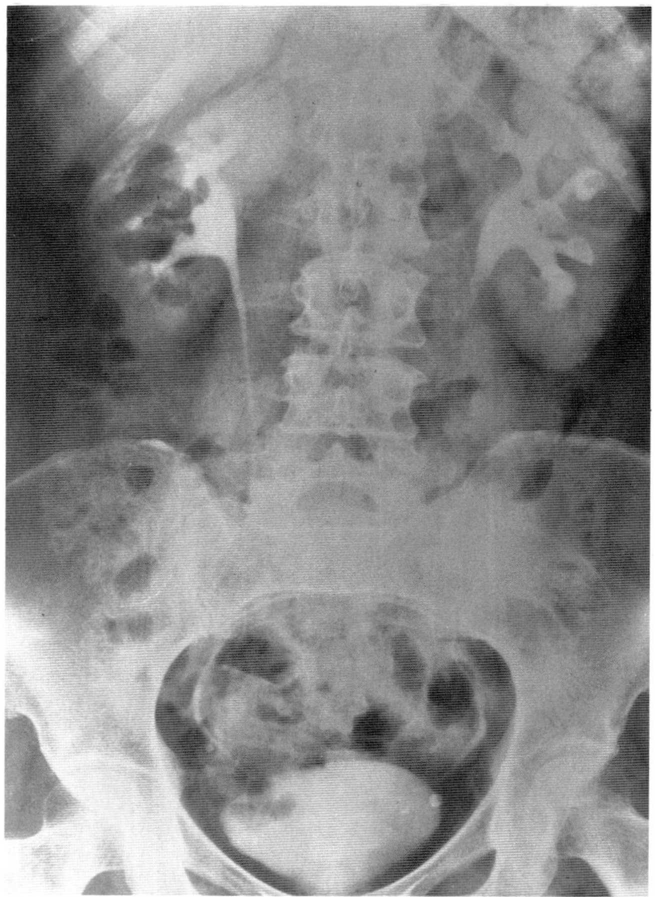

Fig. 73. Case 25. Excretory urogram in a child with thrombocytopenia, revealing a discrete mass effect in the outer portion of the left kidney

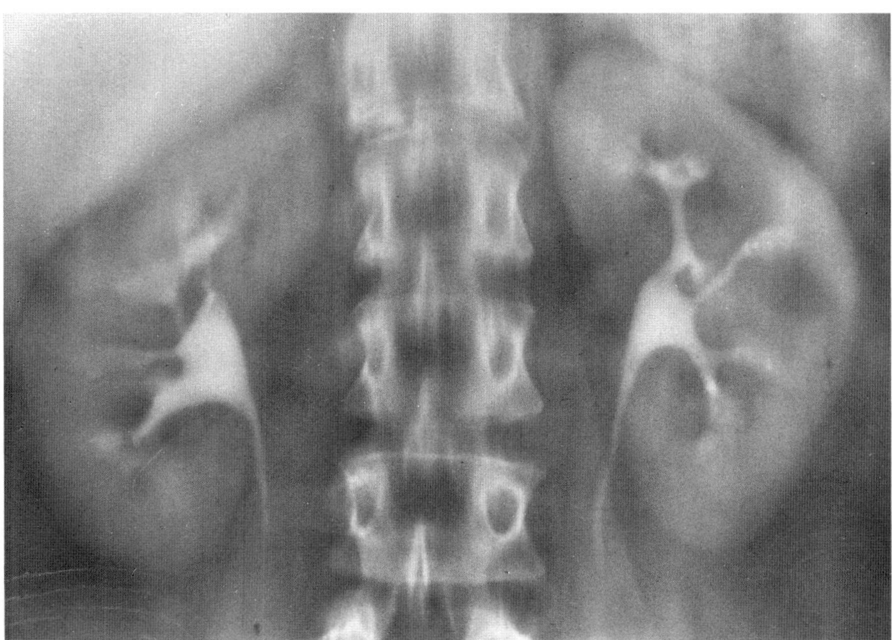

Fig. 74. Case 25. Nephrotomogram. Note a mass effect in the outer middle third of the left kidney. A neoplasm was suspected

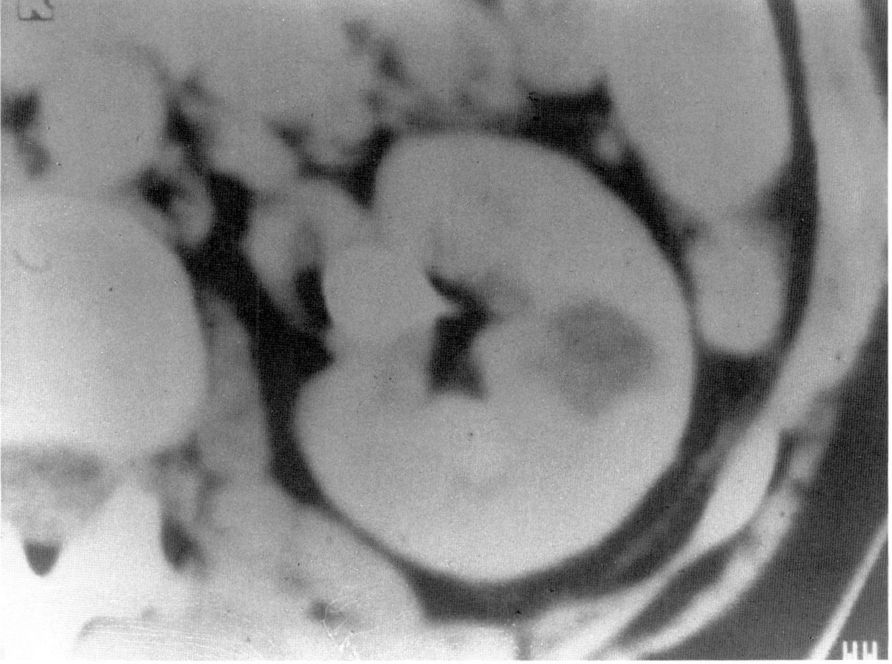

Fig. 75. Case 25. CT of the left kidney showing a mass which does not enhance

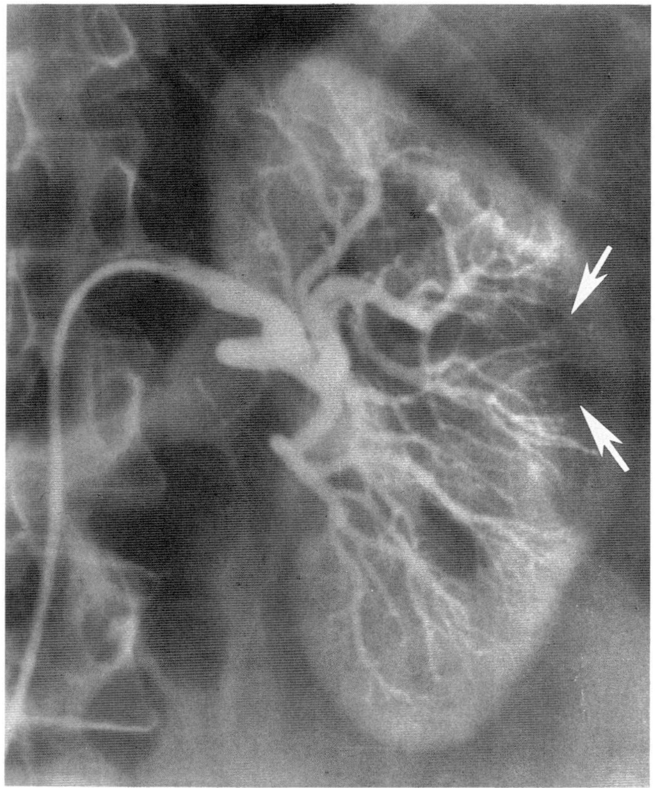

Fig. 76. Case 25. Selective left renal arteriogram. Note absence of vascularity at the site of the mass (*arrows*)

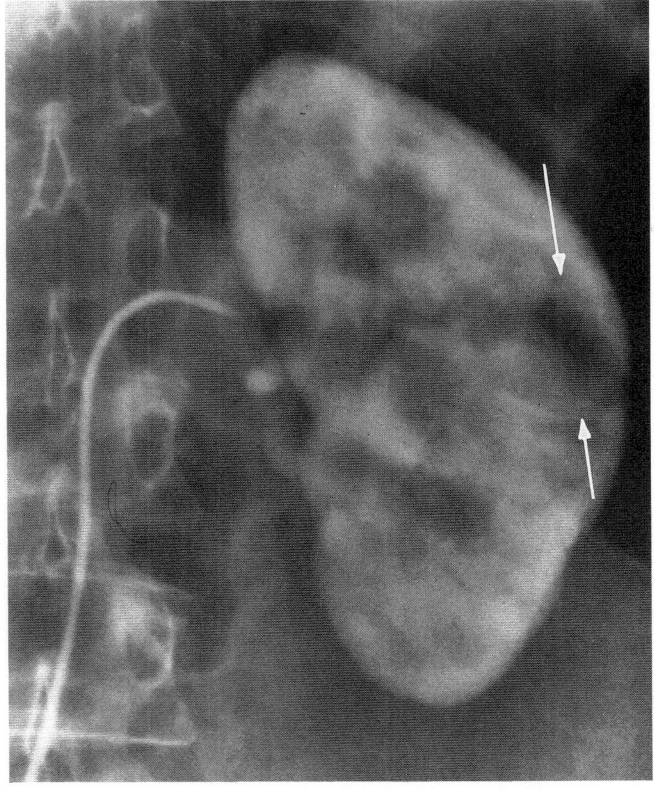

Fig. 77. Case 25. Late parenchymal phase. A mass is seen but there is avascularity (*arrows*)

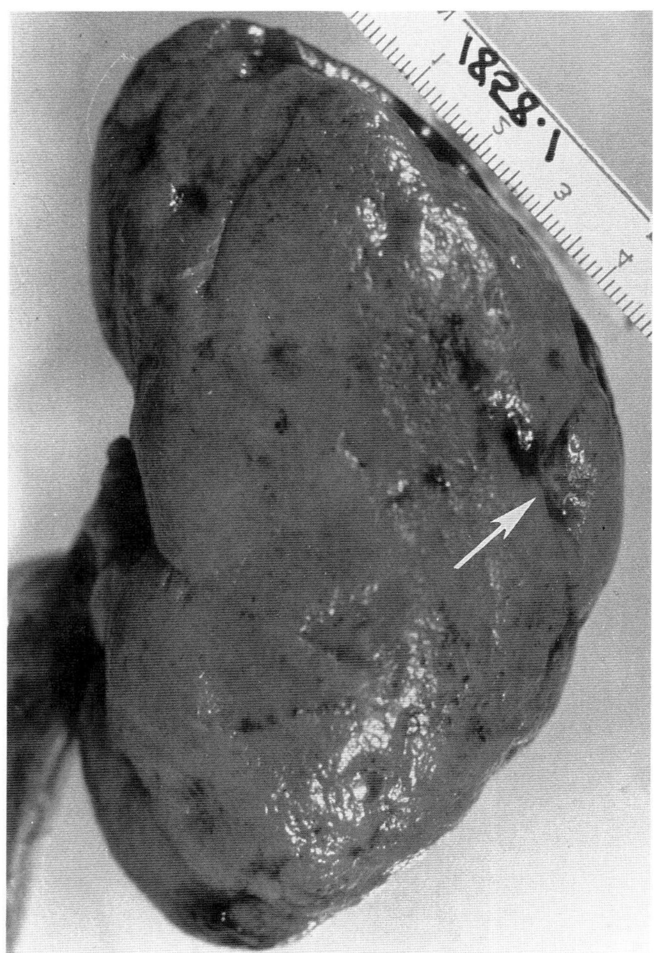

Fig. 78. Case 25. The outer surface of the left kidney shows an area of discrete juxtacortical hemorrhage (*arrow*). On careful sectioning, no tumor was found. Again, an Antopol-Goldman lesion had been responsible for the radiographic findings

The Antopol-Goldman lesion is the name given to a type of renal hematoma that is due to subepithelial bleeding and can simulate a neoplasm.

When there is a history of trauma or a hemorrhagic diathesis and bleeding may be present, the conservative approach is to repeat assessment of the kidney within 1–2 weeks. If a mass has disappeared or has reduced in size, it can be retrospectively interpreted as having represented a hematoma, particularly if ultrasonography, CT, and MRI, as well as arteriography, fail to demonstrate evidence of a neoplasm. It is true that 5%–10% of neoplasms of the kidney show hypovascularity (particularly papillary and transitional cell carcinomas); however, with a history of a bleeding diathesis or trauma, the possibility of a hematoma should always be entertained.

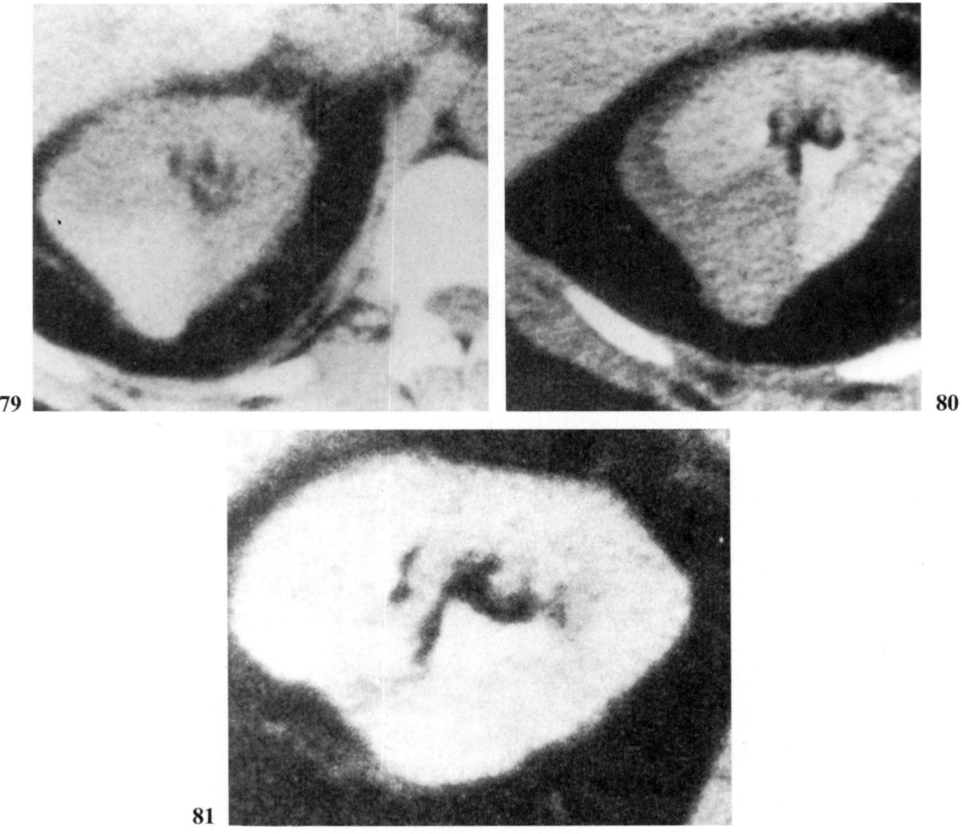

Fig. 79. Case 26. Unenhanced CT scan in a patient with hemorrhagic infarct simulating a renal neoplasm. A renal mass is seen bulging dorsally

Fig. 80. Case 26. Enhanced CT scan

Fig. 81. Case 26. Repeat CT 6 months later shows a scar at the level of the mass. This is another pitfall in the interpretation of a renal mass

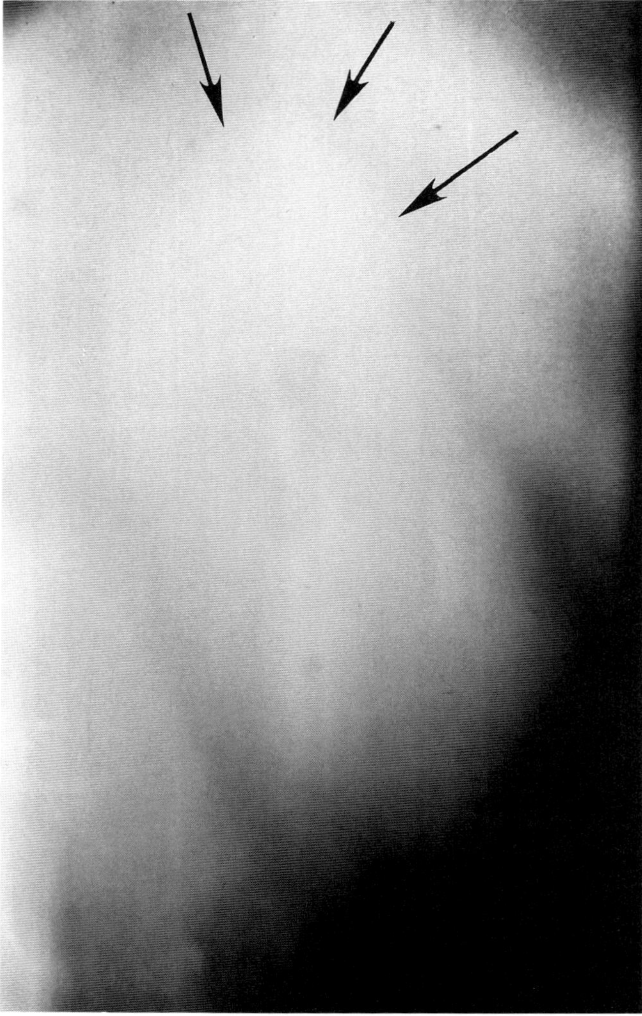

Fig. 82. Case 27. This patient presented with a mass effect (*arrows*) at the upper pole of the left kidney

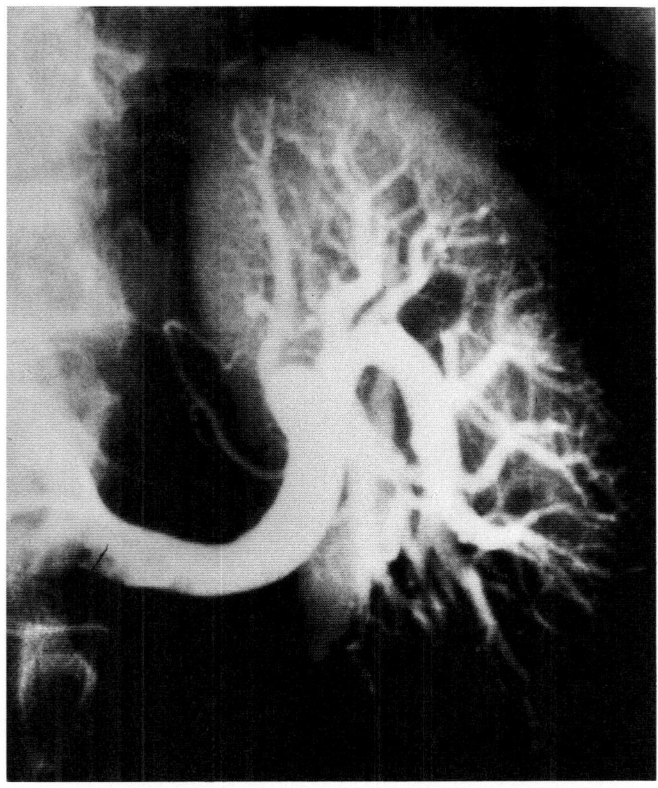

Fig. 83. Case 27. Selective left renal arteriogram, frontal projection, which fails to demonstrate any evidence of a mass

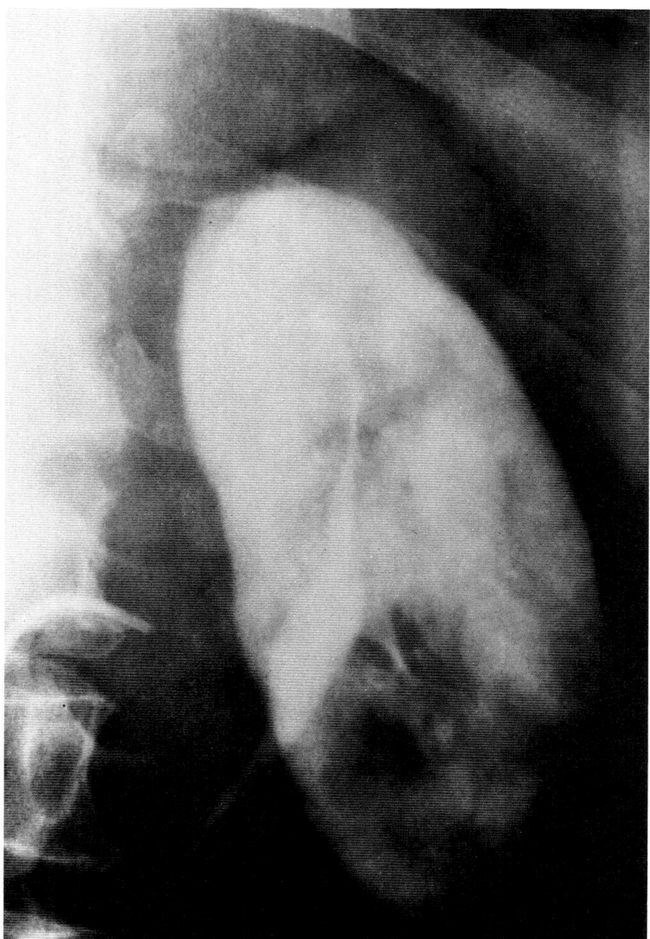

Fig. 84. Case 27. Late phase of selective left renal arteriography. There is slight elongation of the infundibulum to the upper calyces but no definite mass is seen within the kidney. A density is noted, however, adjacent to the upper pole of the left kidney

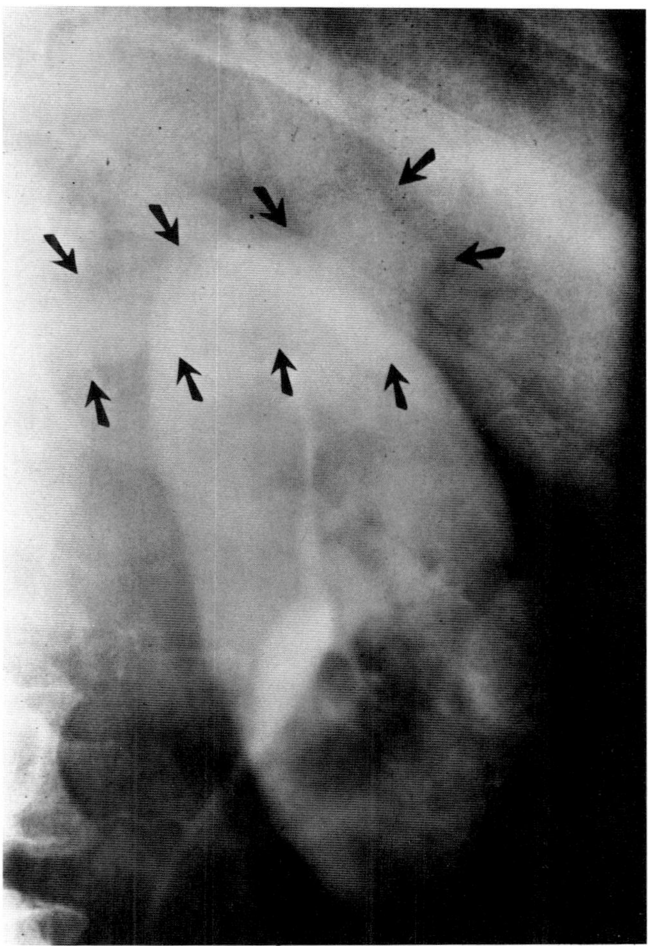

Fig. 85. Case 27. Venous phase of a celiac injection. The splenic vein is opacified as well as the mass (*arrows*). The radiologist interpreted this mass as a pseudotumor caused by a bulbous splenic vein, and even published his observation

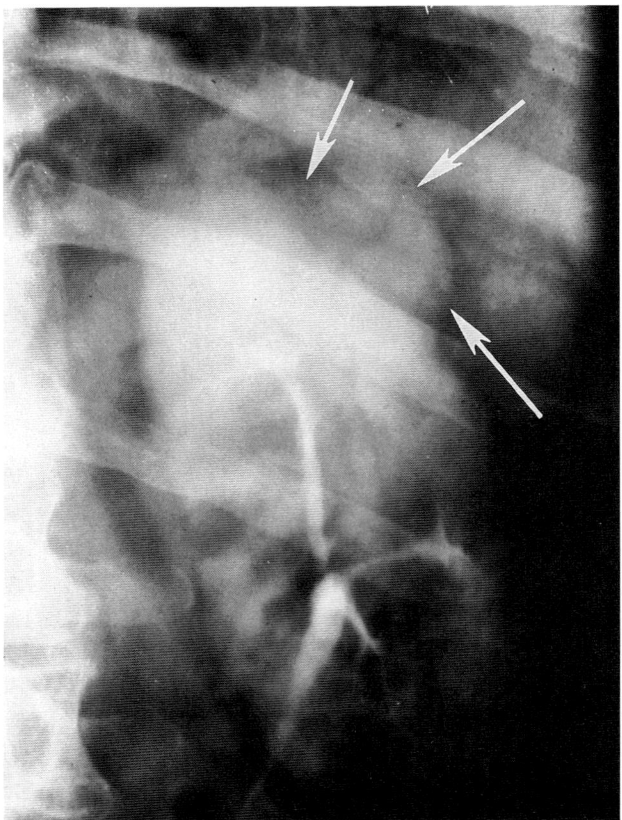

Fig. 86. Case 27. Repeat urogram performed when the patient came to Florida 2 years later, complaining of hematuria. Enlargement of the upper pole of the left kidney (*arrows*) and more elongation of the infundibulum of the left upper calyces are now evident

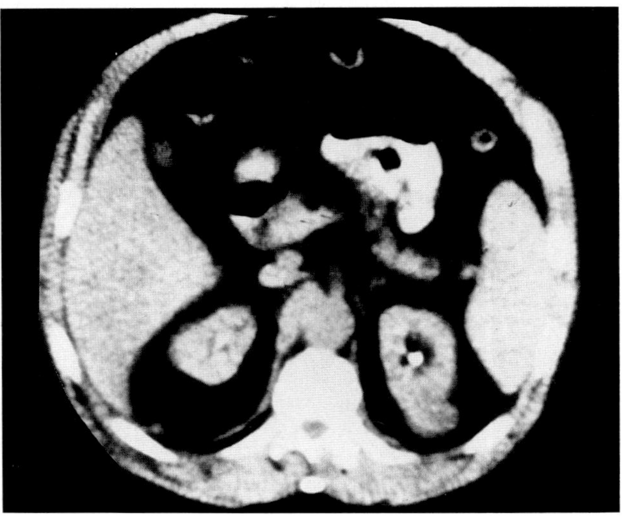

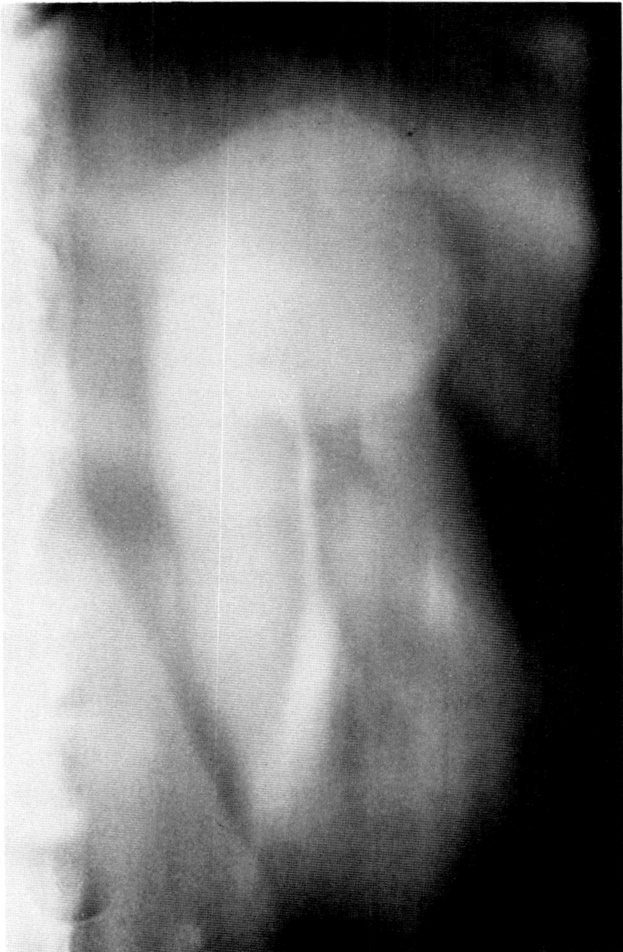

Fig. 87. Case 27. Nephrotomogram in the oblique projection now reveals a large mass within the upper pole of the left kidney

◄

Fig. 88. Case 27. CT examination. Note the neoplasm in the dorsal aspect of the left kidney. At surgery, the mass proved to be a renal carcinoma. This carcinoma could have been suspected 2 years earlier if CT had been performed at that time, or if oblique arteriograms had been obtained. This observation is made through that very important instrument called the retrospectoscope!

There are various forms of renal cystic diseases (see Table 1, Appendix). Multilocular cystic nephroma (MLCN) may be defined as "an uncommon renal *neoplasm* characterized by a well-circumscribed encapsulated mass that contains multiple noncommunicating fluid-filled locules." Like nephroblastoma, MLCN derives from the metanephric blastema. It was first described in 1892, since which time 158 cases have been reported, albeit under a variety of synonyms (see Table 2, Appendix).

Clinical Findings. MLCN shows a bimodal incidence that is sex related. Of male cases, 89% are in those aged between 3 months and 4 years, while 73% of female cases are in adults aged 40–50 years. The symptoms vary according to age: an abdominal mass is the characteristic presenting feature in children, whereas in adults hematuria and abdominal pain are typical. In most cases a solitary cyst is present, but there may be multiple or bilateral cysts. The most common location is the lower pole. Growth may occur slowly, over years, or rapidly, within months.

Radiologic Findings. See Table 3, Appendix.

Treatment is by nephrectomy. Local recurrence and metastasis are uncommon (having occurred in only 4 of the 158 reported cases).

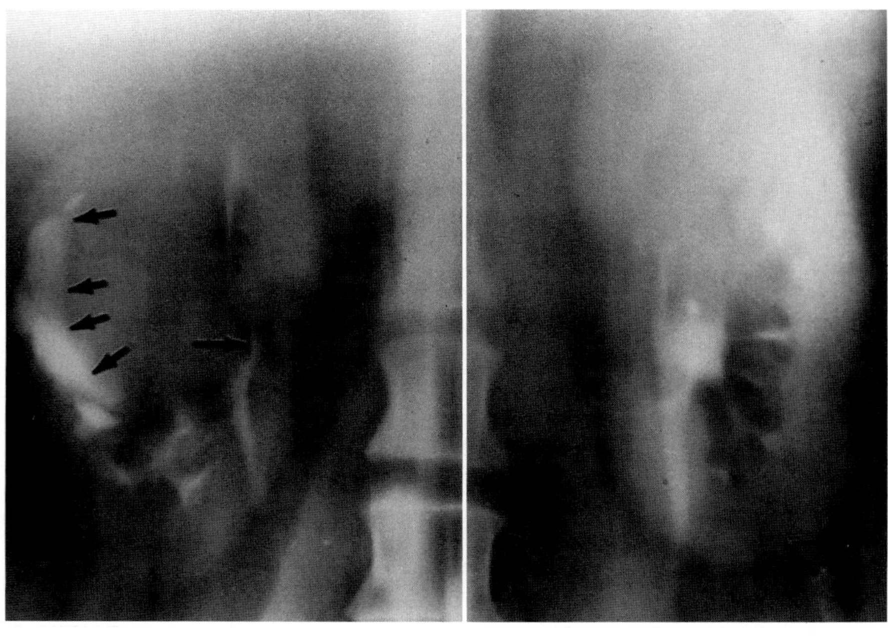

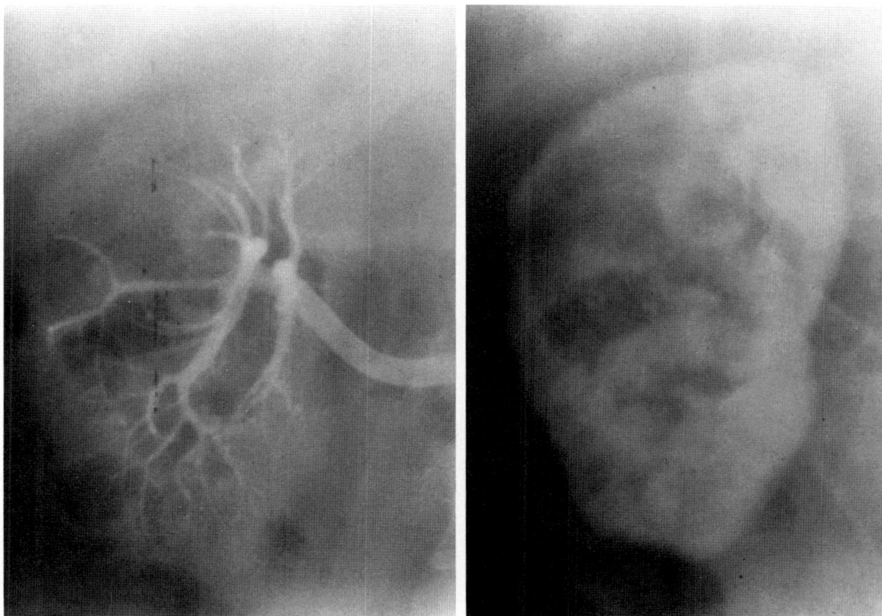

Fig. 90 a, b. Case 28. Selective right renal arteriography, early arterial phase (**a**) and parenchymal phase (**b**). Both phases reveal an avascular irregular mass in the central portion of the right kidney. At this time I thought the patient had a necrotic carcinoma of the right kidney. I asked the patient to lie on his stomach and then I punctured the mass. A yellow fluid was retrieved; the cytologic findings later proved negative and there was no evidence of fat

◄───

Fig. 89. Case 28. Tomogram of a 68-year-old man with a history of gouty arthropathy and with elevated BUN and back pain. A mass, causing compression of the right middle calyces and of the upper right ureter (*arrows*), was found in the central portion of the right kidney. A dear friend of mine, a Professor of Urology, wanted to "explore" the patient. His reasoning was that if this was a neoplasm, he would perform a nephrectomy, while if it was a cyst, he would decompress the cyst. However, I felt that if this was a benign process, removal of the right kidney would worsen the kidney function in view of the fact that the patient already had elevated BUN, probably due to gouty nephropathy. The patient consulted with me and I performed selective right renal arteriography

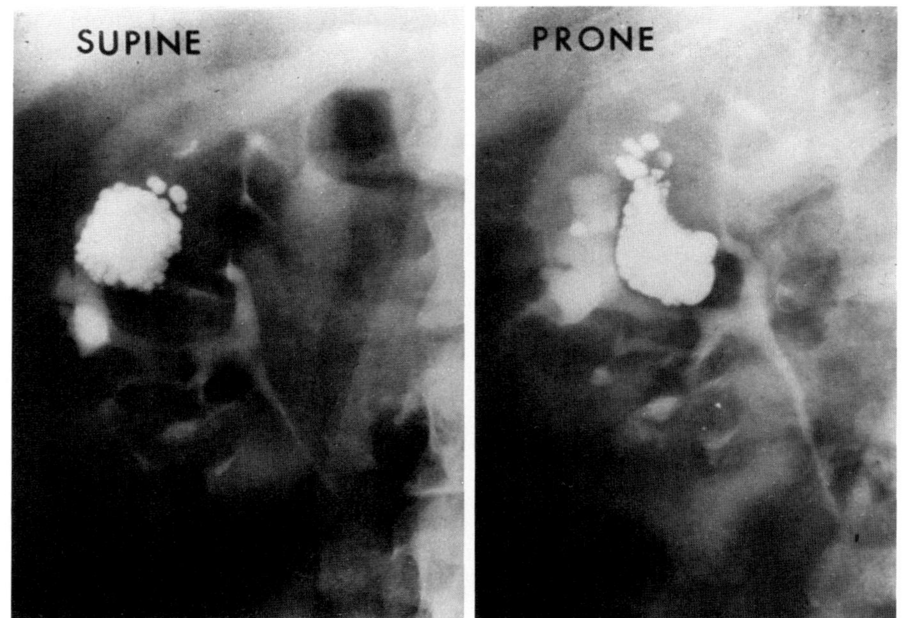

Fig. 91 a, b. Case 28. Films obtained with the patient in the supine and prone positions following injection of contrast medium (Pantopaque), which dispersed irregularly

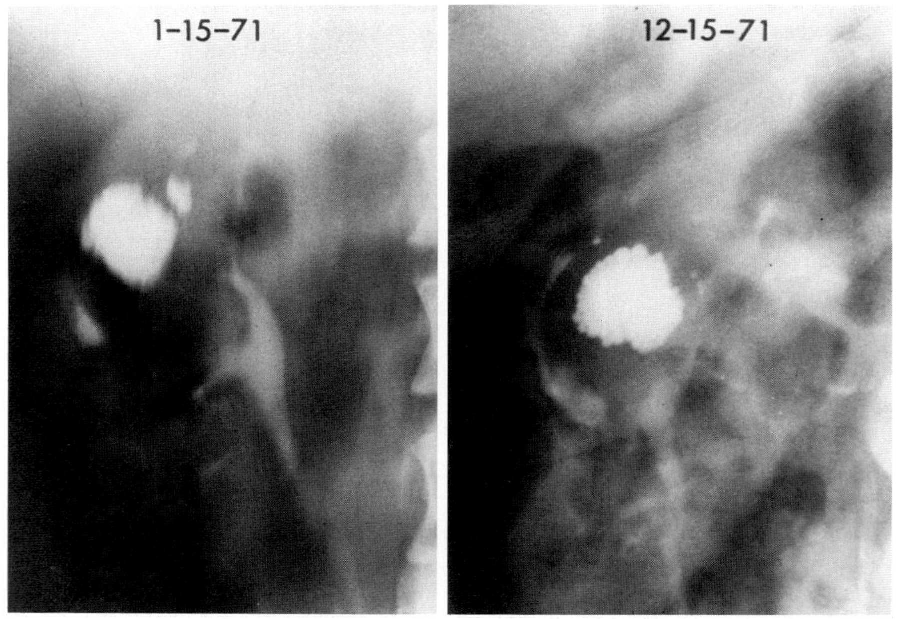

Fig. 92 a, b. Case 28. Comparative urograms showing a reduction in the size of the mass at almost 1 year of follow-up. The patient was followed up for 15 years and there was no evidence of any growth of the mass. Retrospectively, the constellation of findings suggested the presence of a multilocular cystic nephroma. I still have a Rolex watch given to me by this grateful patient!

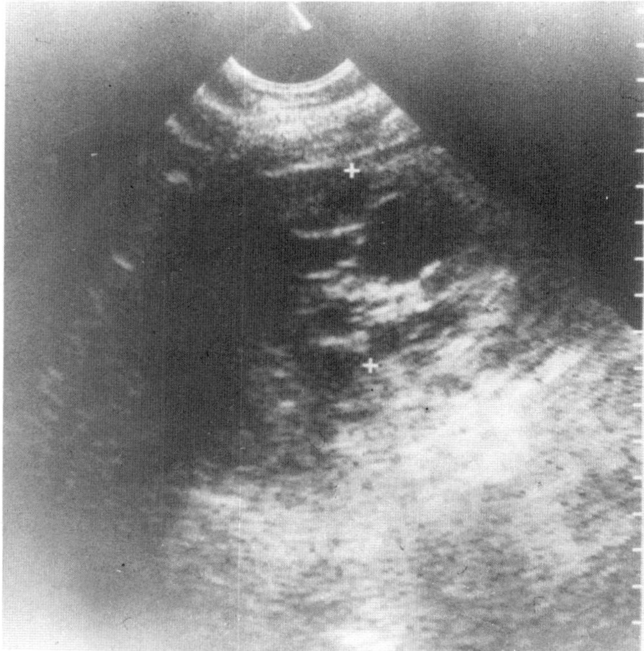

Fig. 93. Case 29. Ultrasonogram showing cystic and solid components of a mass in the outer portion of the right kidney

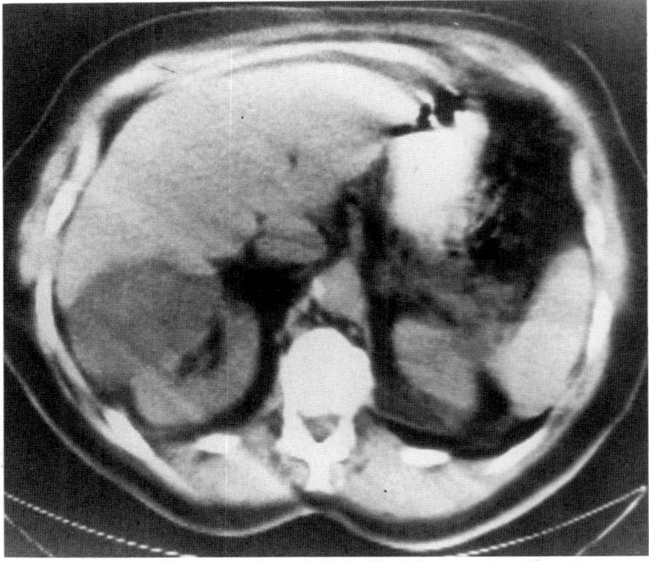

Fig. 94. Case 29. CT of the right kidney showing the exophytic mass

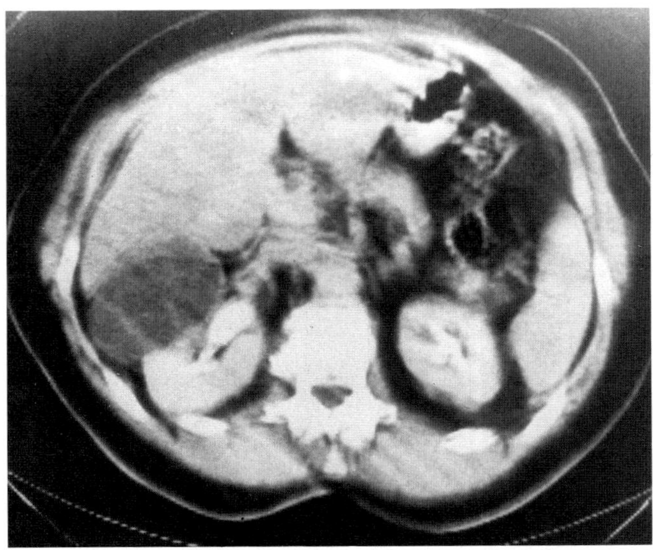

Fig. 95. Case 29. Enhanced CT. Note that most of the mass appears to be avascular

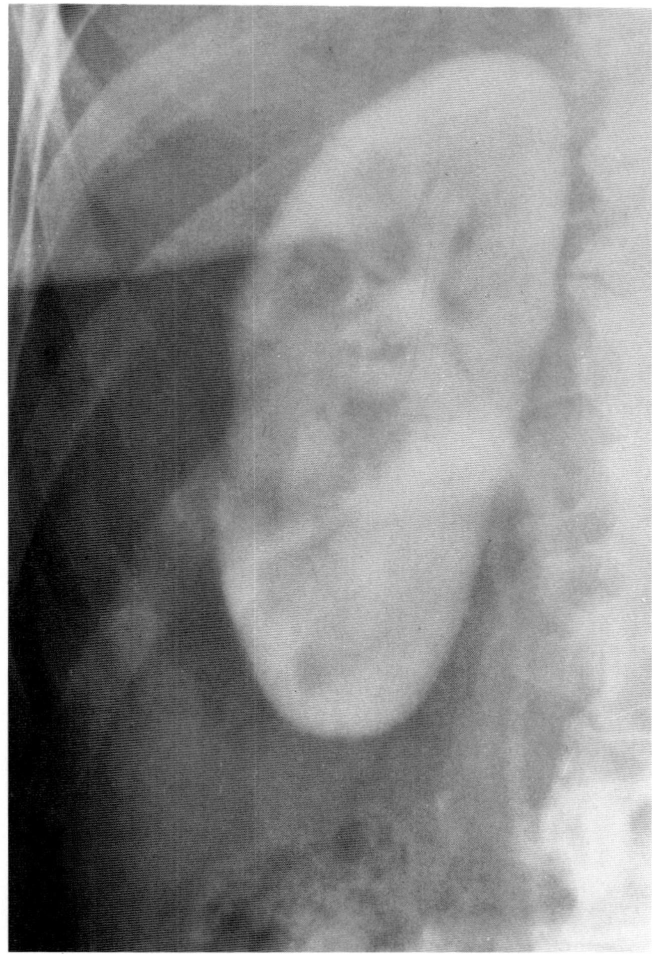

Fig. 96. Case 29. Selective right renal arteriogram, late phase. Note avascular mass in the outer aspect of the right kidney. The mass was punctured and clear fluid was retrieved. Contrast medium was injected and dispersed in an irregular fashion

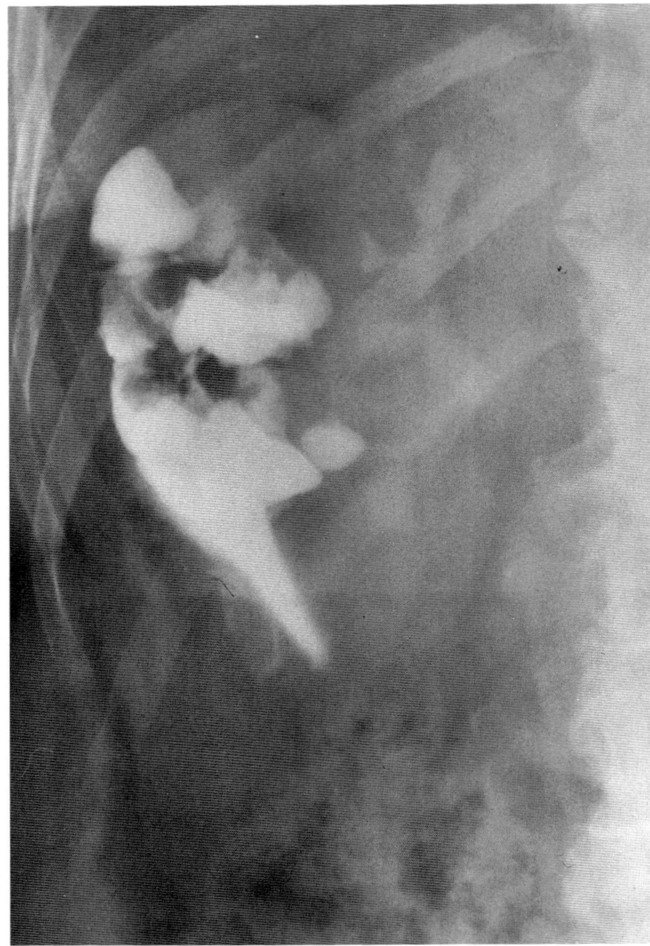

Fig. 97. Case 29. Oblique view of the right kidney following the injection of contrast medium. Note irregular dispersion of the contrast. At surgery, no tumor was found. Histologically, this proved to be another example of a multilocular cystic nephroma

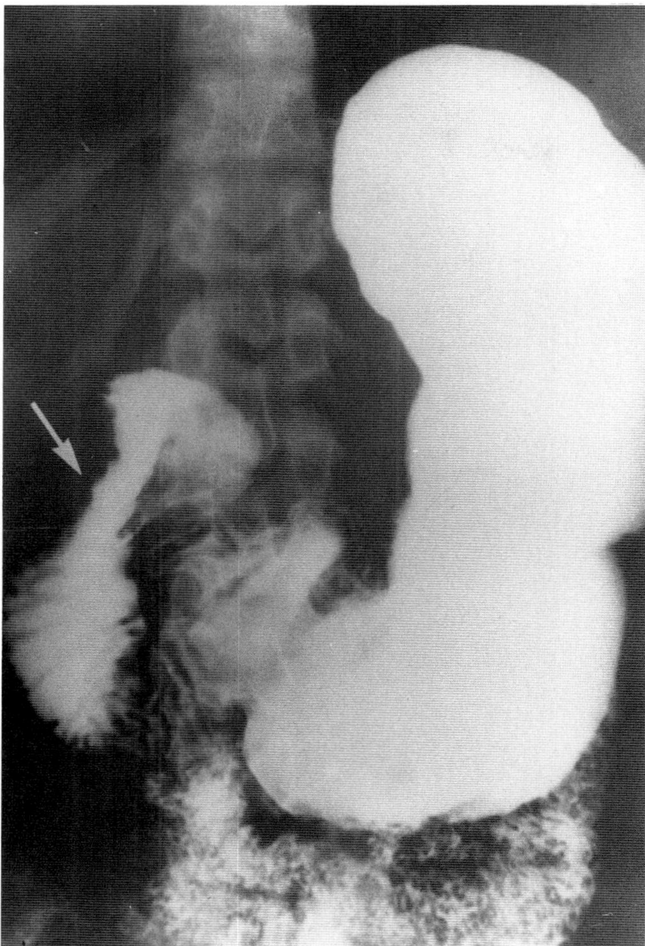

Fig. 98. Case 30. An upper gastrointestinal series in an 18-year-old woman with a 2-week history of right upper quadrant pain and tenderness revealed a mass compressing the second part of the duodenum (*arrow*). Physical examination had suggested the presence of the mass, and a bruit had also been noted. There was no hematuria, no hypertension, and no history of fever. Biliary tract pathology was suspected

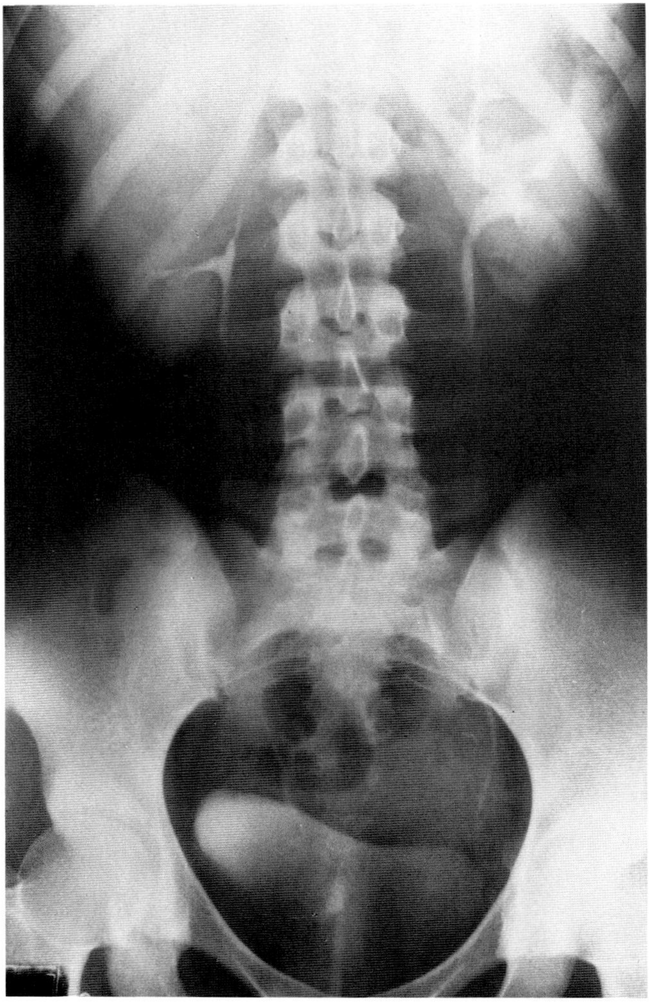

Fig. 99. Case 30. Excretory urogram revealing a mass in the upper portion of the right kidney, with downward displacement of the right renal pelvis

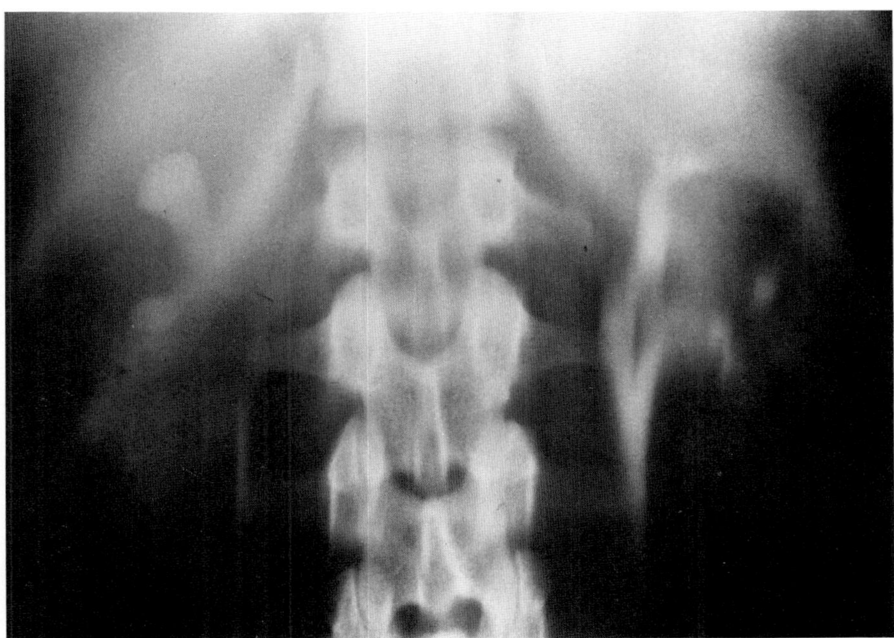

Fig. 100. Case 30. Nephrotomogram showing dilated right upper calyx and a mass in the upper two-thirds of the right kidney

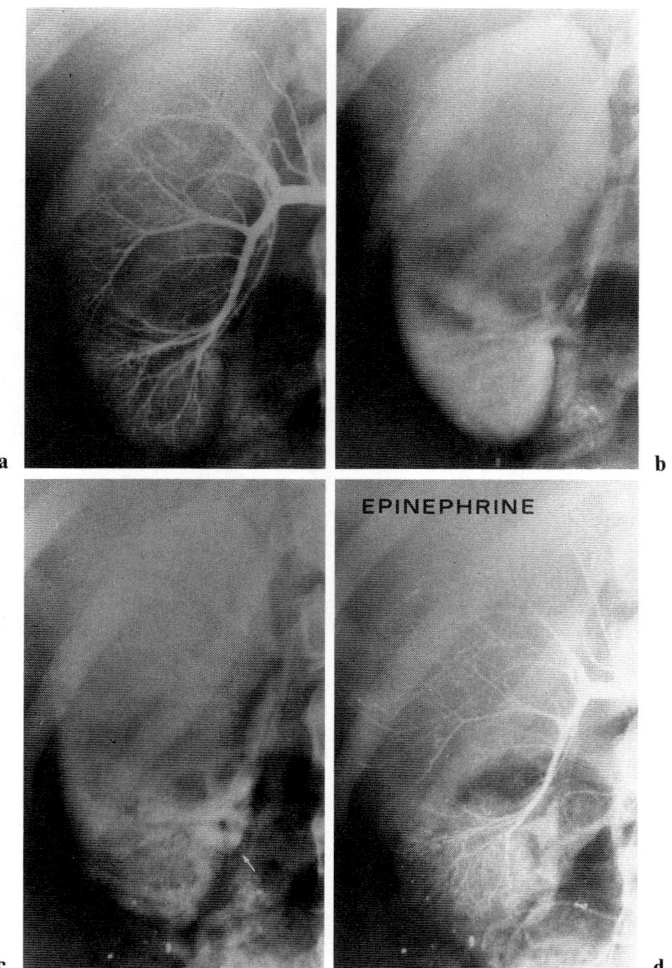

Fig. 101 a–d. Case 30. Selective right renal arteriogram without (**a–c**) and following (**d**) epinephrine injection shows a mass in the upper two-thirds of the right kidney with minimal neovascularity. Note that the vessels within the mass remain opacified after the injection of epinephrine into the right renal artery. Note also evidence of obstruction of the right renal vein as manifested by lack of opacification of the right renal vein and collateral veins in the medial lower portion of the right kidney. Neoplasia was suspected extending beyond the kidney and affecting the second part of the duodenum. At surgery, no neoplasia was found. The right kidney was removed

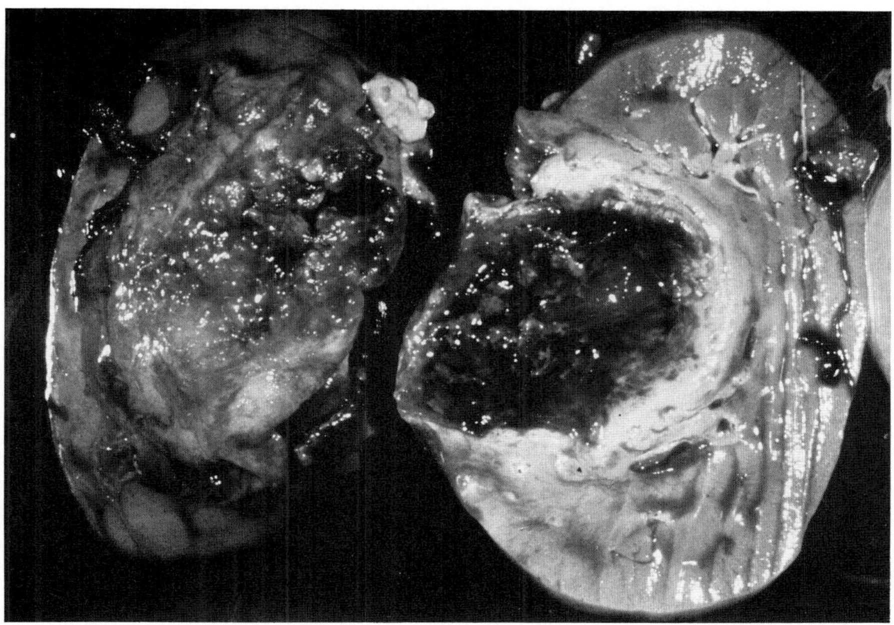

Fig. 102. Case 30. Open specimen of the right kidney. Histologically, this proved to be a case of xanthogranulomatous pyelonephritis

In cases of xanthogranulomatous pyelonephritis, intravenous pyelography reveals absent or decreased kidney function and staghorn calculus (or stricture) obstruction. The kidney is usually enlarged (either uniformly or asymmetrically) and the kidney outline may be poorly defined. Angiography is inconclusive, i.e., vascularity may be increased or decreased, there may be a positive or a negative response to epinephrine, and veins may be patent or obstructed.

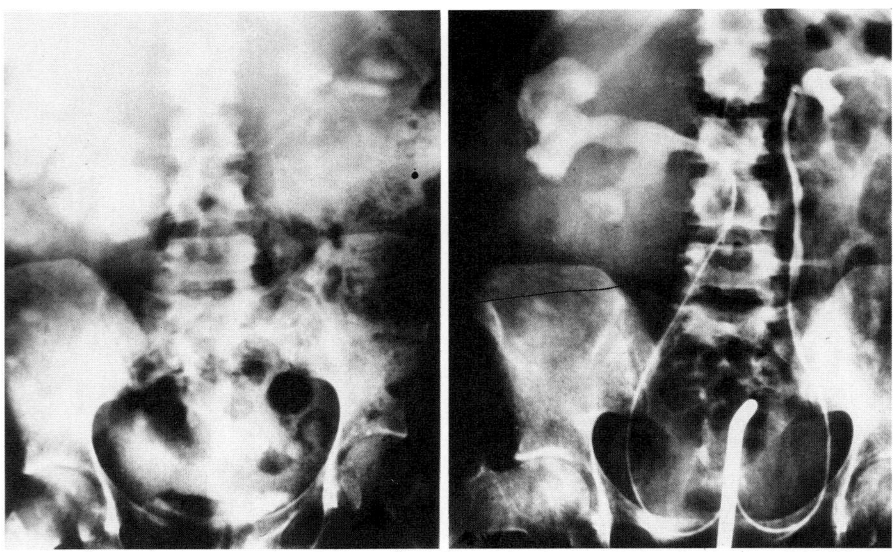

Fig. 103a, b. Case 31. **a** Excretory urogram in a young woman with high blood pressure, evidence of renal failure, and palpable abdominal masses in the right upper quadrant and both flanks. The urogram shows a dilated and distorted pelvocalyceal system. Discrete densities are scattered throughout the innominate bone. **b** Bilateral retrograde pyelogram showing no evidence of obstructive uropathy but a dilated, distorted pelvocalyceal system. Again, blastic areas are visualized throughout the innominate bone

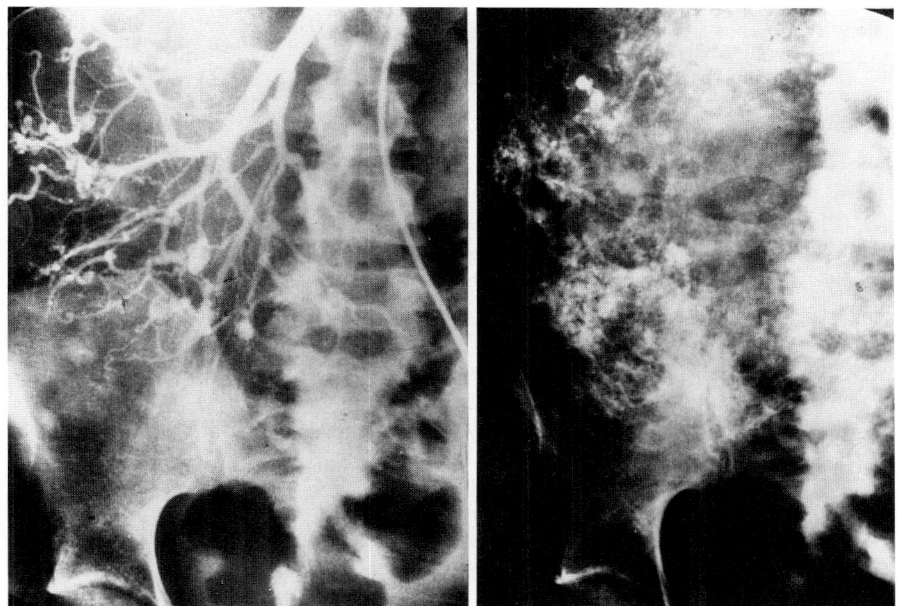

Fig. 104 a, b. Case 31. Selective right renal arteriogram: **a** arterial phase, **b** parenchymal phase. Note aneurysms arising from interlobar renal arteries. Marked hypervascularity is noted within the right kidney, particularly in the parenchymal phase. The patient had been explored at another institution and the erroneous diagnosis of polycystic disease had been made. The urologist had failed to recognize the classic skin and radiographic features of tuberous sclerosis. A second abdominal exploration was performed and biopsies of the kidney showed no evidence of tumor. The typical histological findings of angiomyolipomas were noted

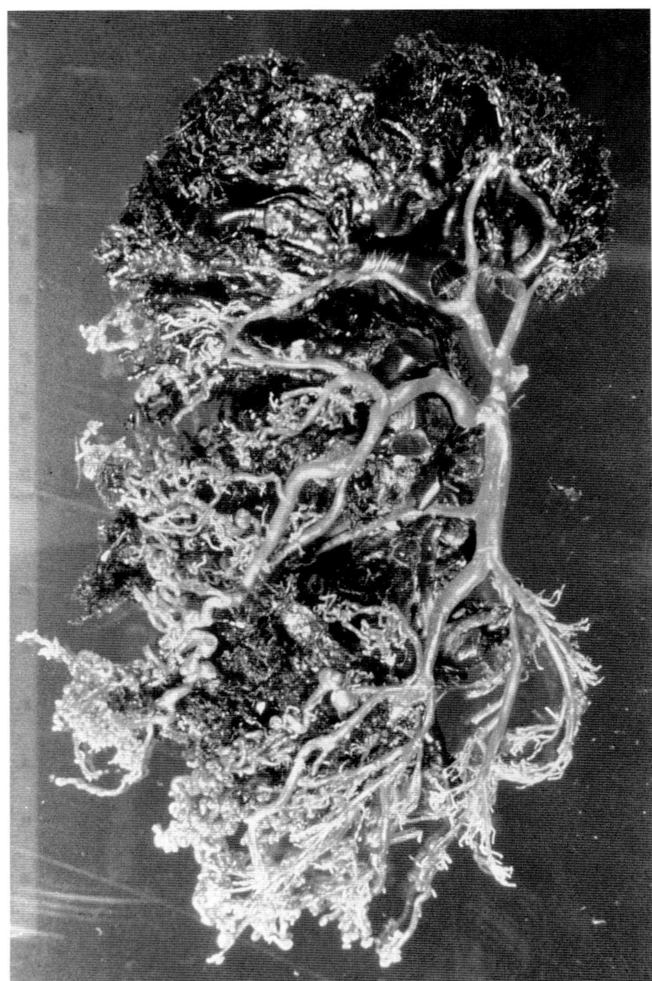

Fig. 105. Cast corrosion preparation from a patient with angiomyolipomas of the right kidney. Note macroaneurysms arising from interlobar renal arteries. The size of the aneurysms and the absence of arterial obstruction and of arteriovenous communications rule out the possibilities of polyarteritis nodosa and necrotizing angiitis. I believe a presentation such as this, with macroaneurysms arising from the interlobar renal arteries, is pathognomonic for renal angiomyolipoma

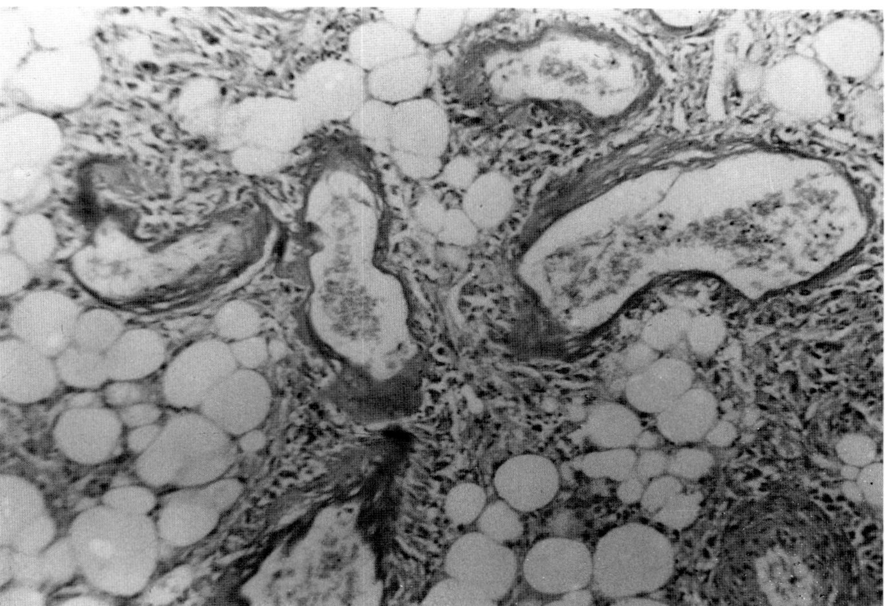

Fig. 106. Histological section of an angiomyolipoma showing increase in number of vessels, fat, and hyperplasia of smooth muscle

In tuberous sclerosis, 80% of patients have bilateral renal angiomyolipomas. I have seen only very few patients with bilateral angiomyolipomas without tuberous sclerosis. Approximately 50% of patients with angiomyolipomas have tuberous sclerosis while the remainder have solitary angiomyolipomas unrelated to tuberous sclerosis

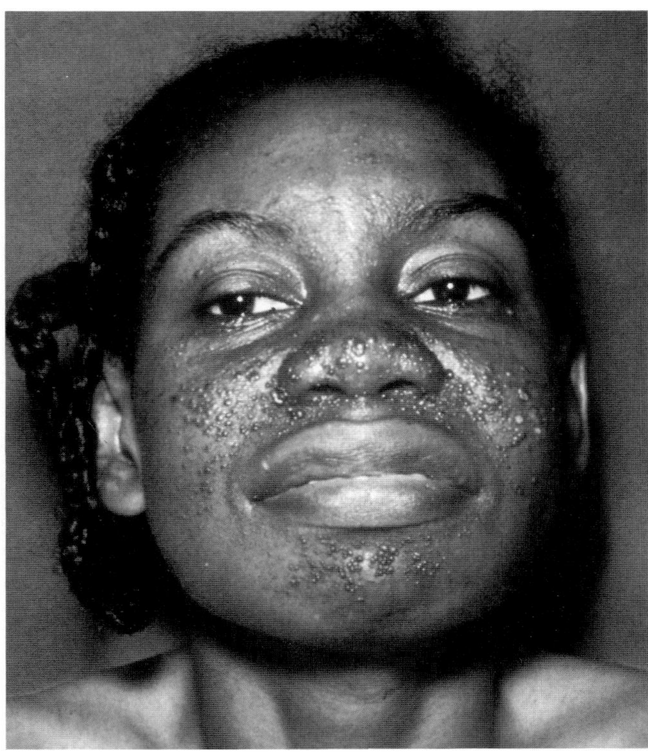

Fig. 107. Photograph of a woman with mental retardation, angiofibromas of the skin (miscalled adenoma sebaceum), and convulsions. This is the so-called epiloia, the clinical triad of tuberous sclerosis

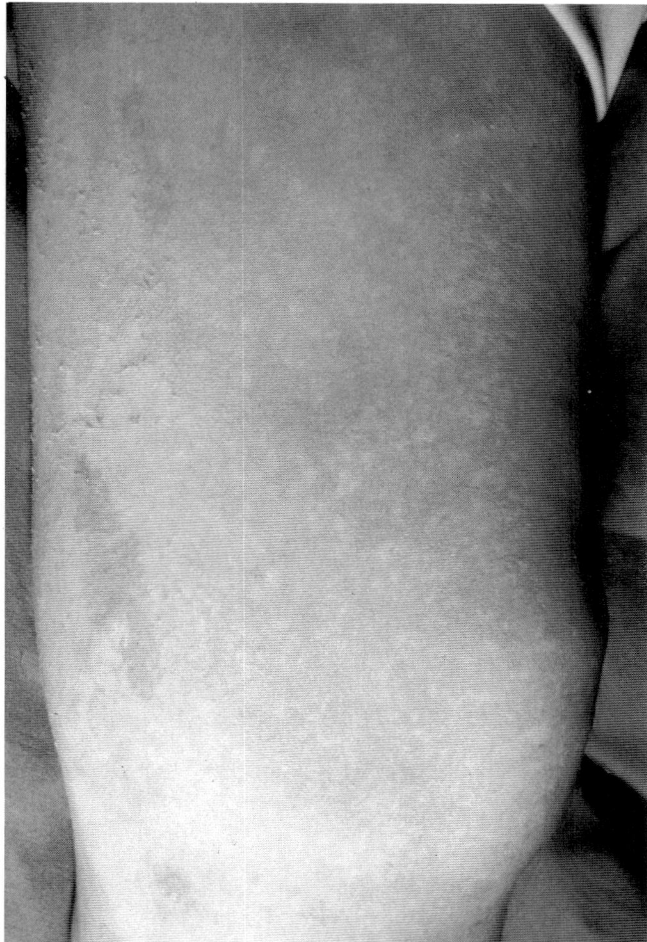

Fig. 108. Café au lait spots in the skin of a patient with tuberous sclerosis

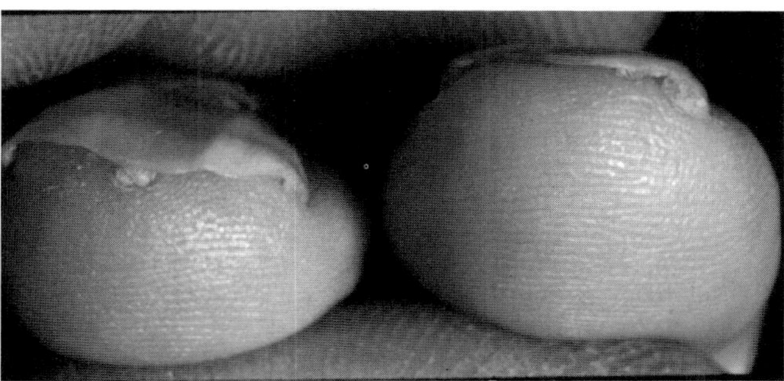

Fig. 109. Subungual fibromas, the pathognomonic clinical signs of tuberous sclerosis with onychodysplasia

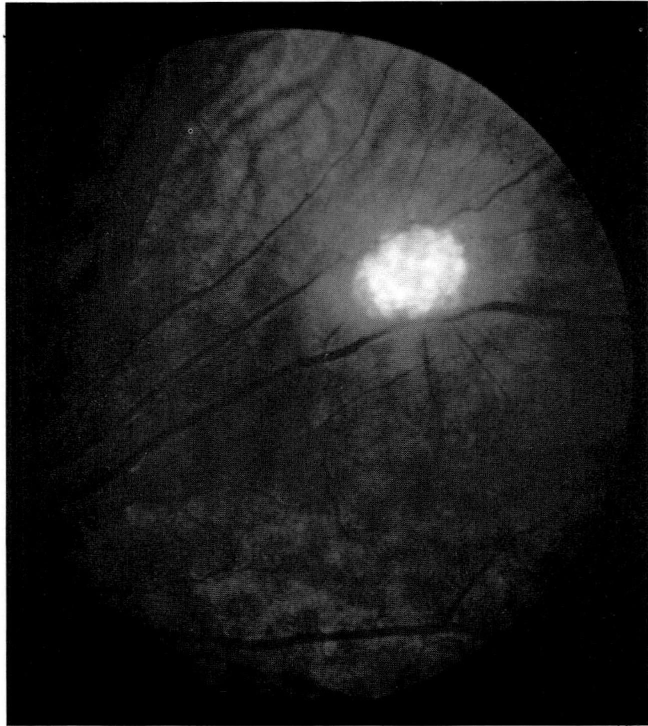

Fig. 110. Phakoma of the retina (yellow plaques), another characteristic feature of tuberous sclerosis

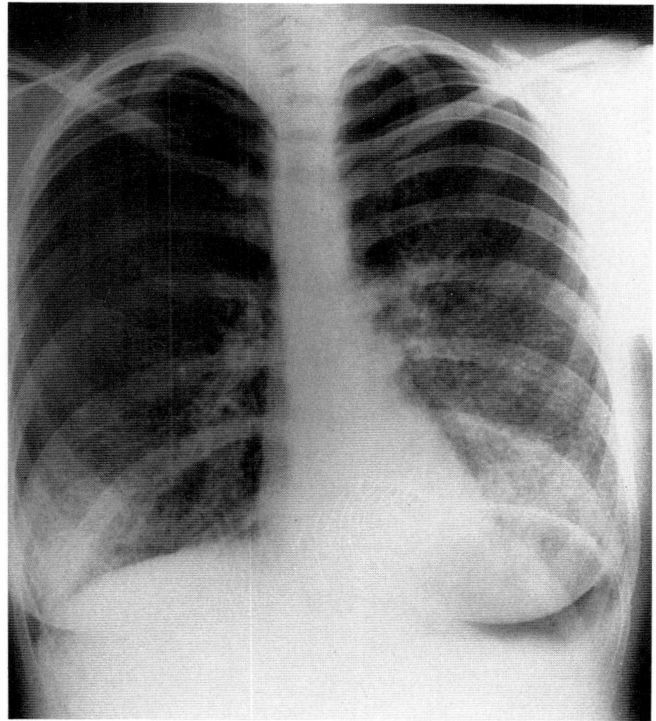

Fig. 111. Case 32. Chest radiograph showing bilateral pneumothorax and a diffuse reticular pattern throughout the lungs in a patient who presented with chest pain

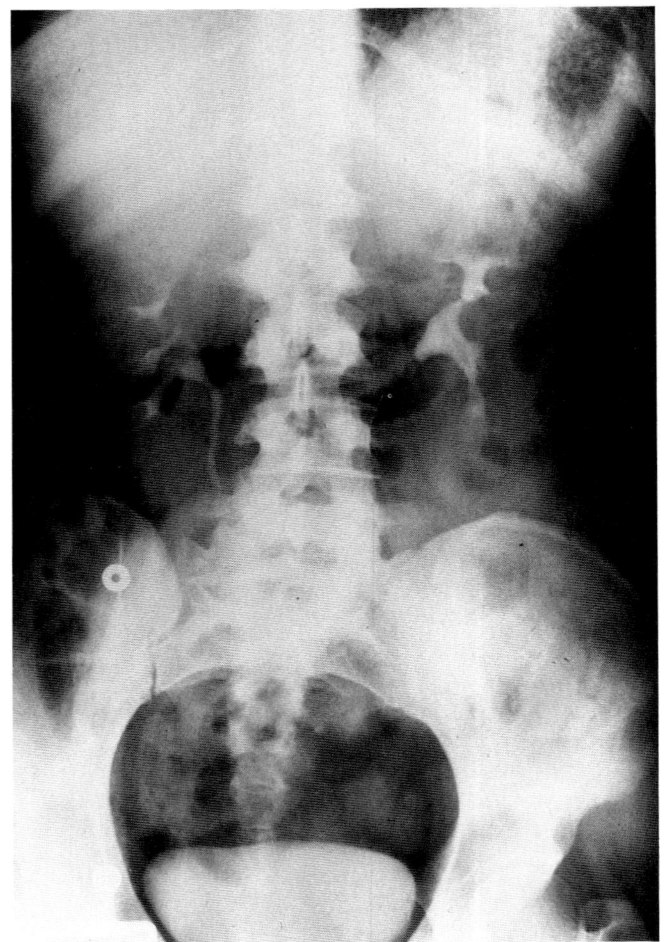

112

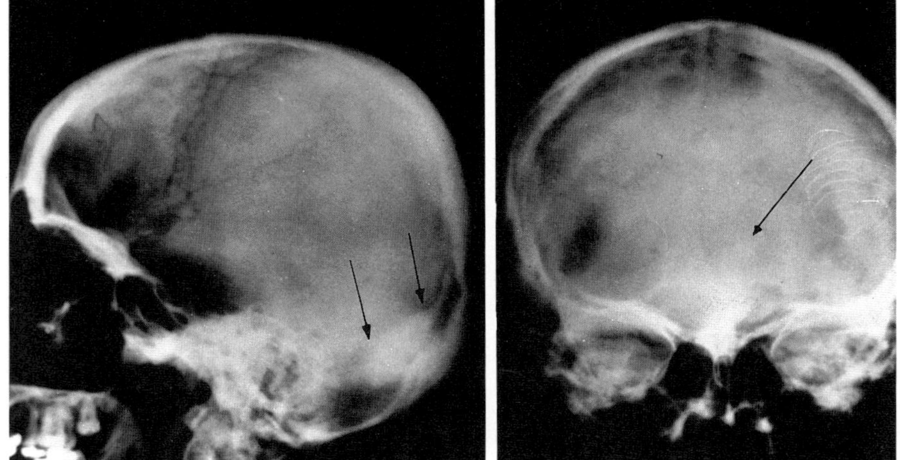

a b

113

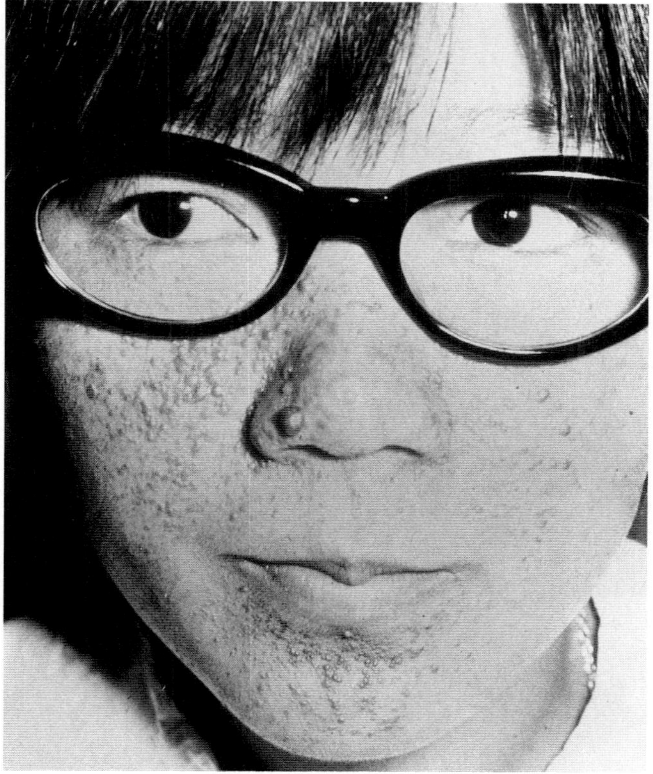

Fig. 114. Case 33. Photograph of Vietnamese girl with cutaneous angiofibromas, also called adenoma sebaceum

◄———

Fig. 112. Case 32. Excretory urogram showing bilaterally enlarged kidneys without distortion of the pelvocalyceal system and no evidence of obstructive uropathy. The initial diagnosis was of an infiltrating process affecting both kidneys. Note sclerotic areas in the ilium and sacrum. The patient was explored and the diagnosis was amended to bilateral angiomyolipomas

Fig. 113 a, b. Case 32. Skull roentgenogram: **a** lateral and **b** frontal projections. Note surface plaques of calcium and calcification of the basal ganglia (*arrows*)

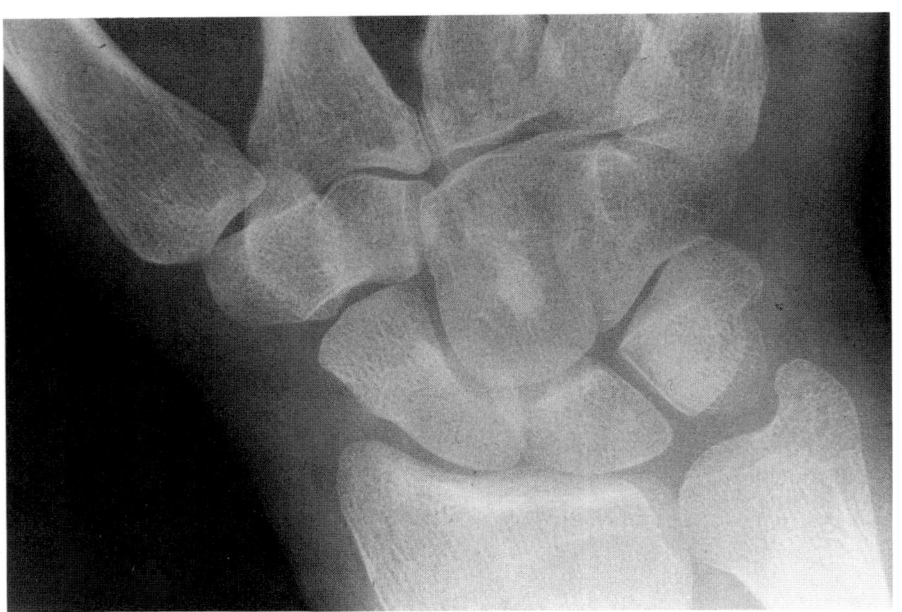

115

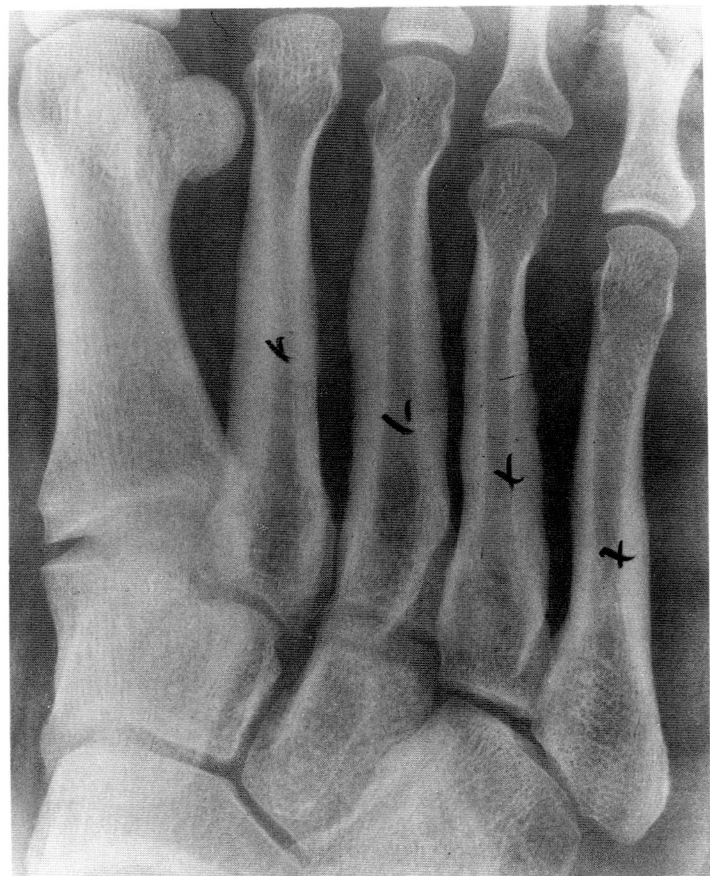

116

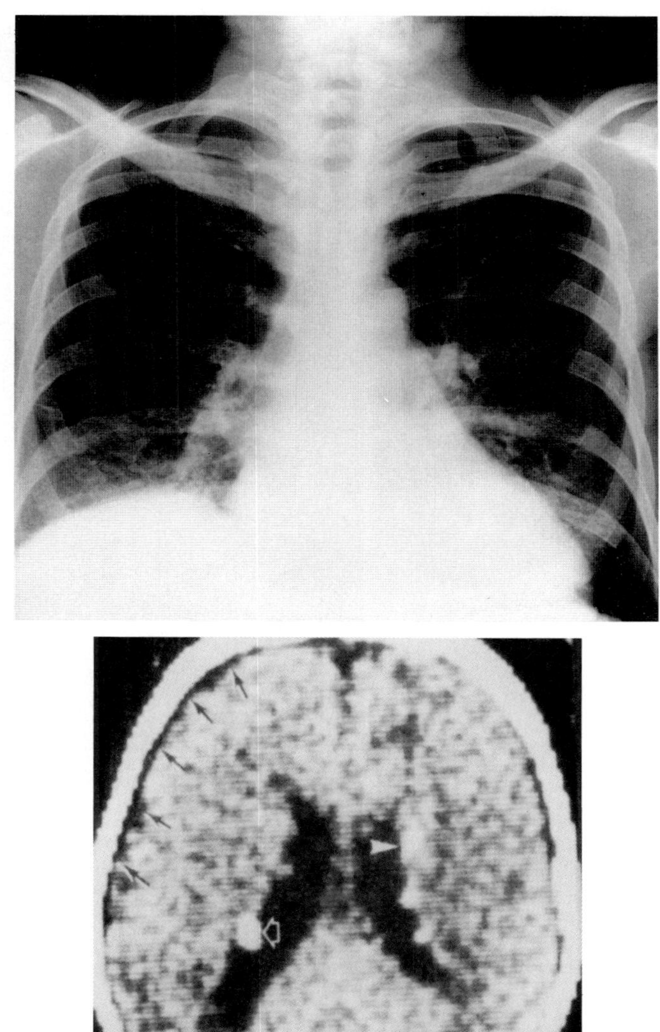

Fig. 117. Case 33. Chest radiograph showing pulmonary hamartomatous changes (bibasilar reticulation) and enlarged left ventricle (secondary to rhabdomyomas)

Fig. 118. Case 33. CT of the brain showing periventricular area of calcifications simulating toxoplasmosis and cytomegalic inclusion disease (*open arrow* and *arrowhead*). There were other areas of calcification in the brain (*arrows*)

Fig. 115. Case 33. Films of the wrist showing sclerotic areas in carpal bones. These are bone islands which are the hamartomas of bone in tuberous sclerosis

Fig. 116. Case 33. Foot: focal cortical thickening, another hamartomatous expression of tuberous sclerosis

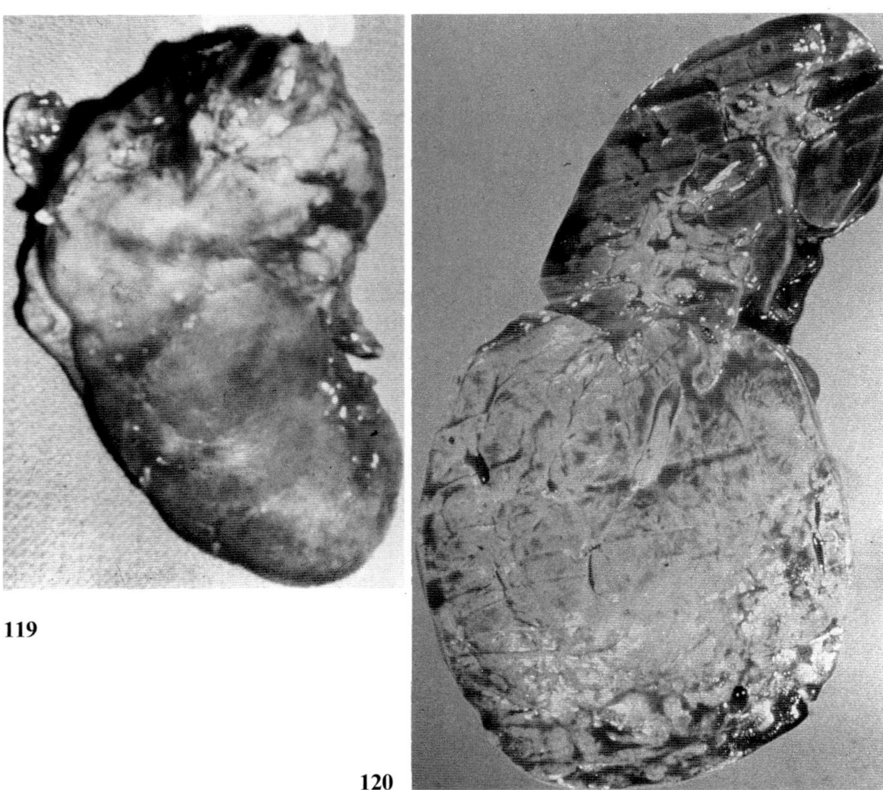

119

120

Fig. 119. Specimen of solitary angiomyolipoma. Note hemorrhagic area in upper pole. At surgery, most solitary angiomyolipomas are believed to represent carcinomas, particularly because of the infiltrating features of the lesion. The angiomatous elements produce the hemorrhagic appearance

Fig. 120. Angiomyolipoma with myomatous elements that predominate. This gives a fleshy appearance to the tumor

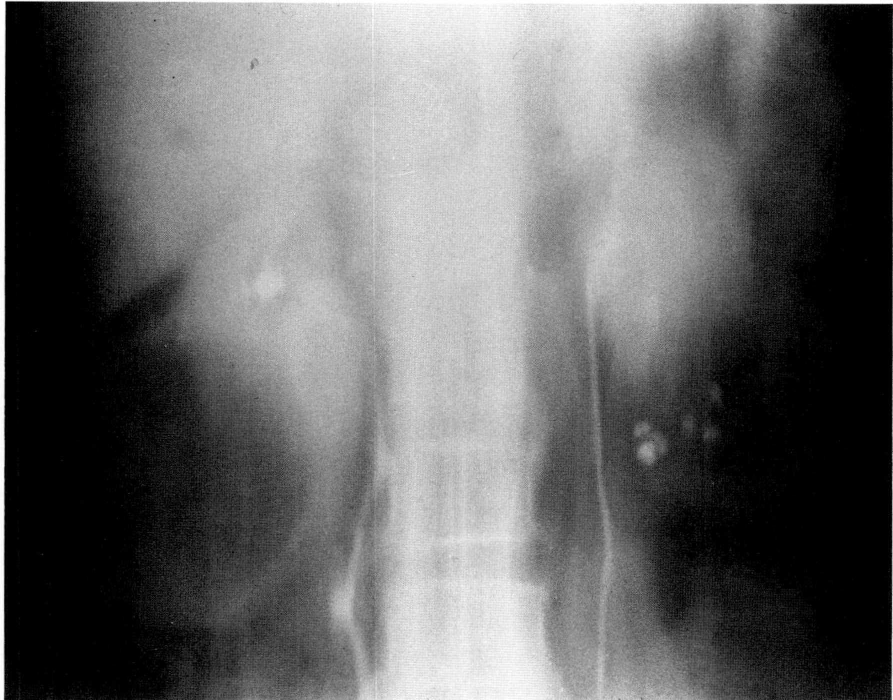

Fig. 121. Case 34. Solitary angiomyolipoma with fatty predominance. This nephrotomogram shows a low density, well-circumscribed mass in the lower pole of the right kidney

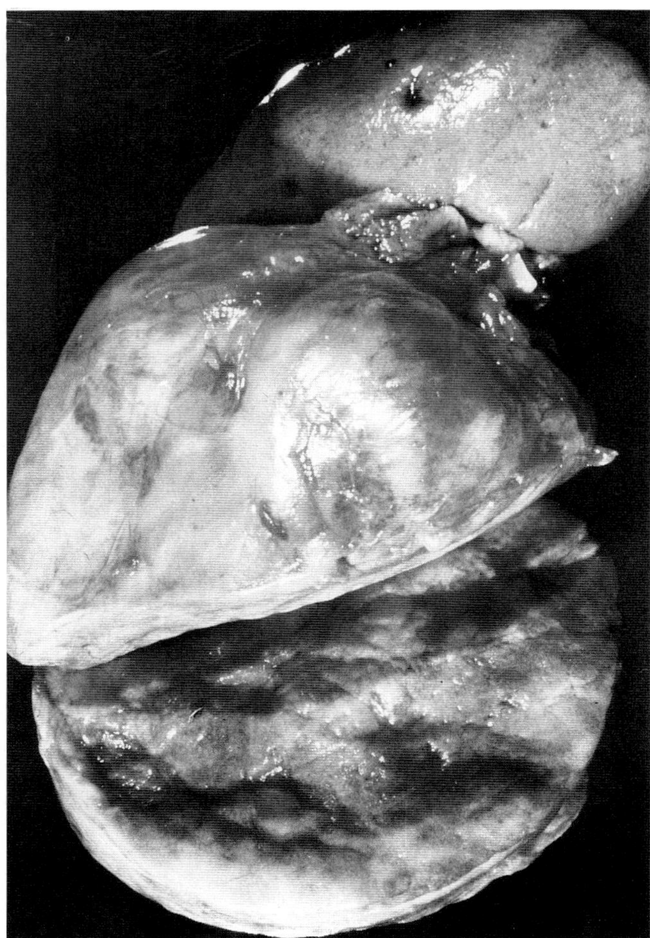

Fig. 122. Specimen of case 34. The lower portion of the right kidney revealed a yellowish appearance. The fatty elements predominate. The angio-, myo-, or lipomatous elements can predominate in angiomyolipomas, the morphological appearance varying accordingly

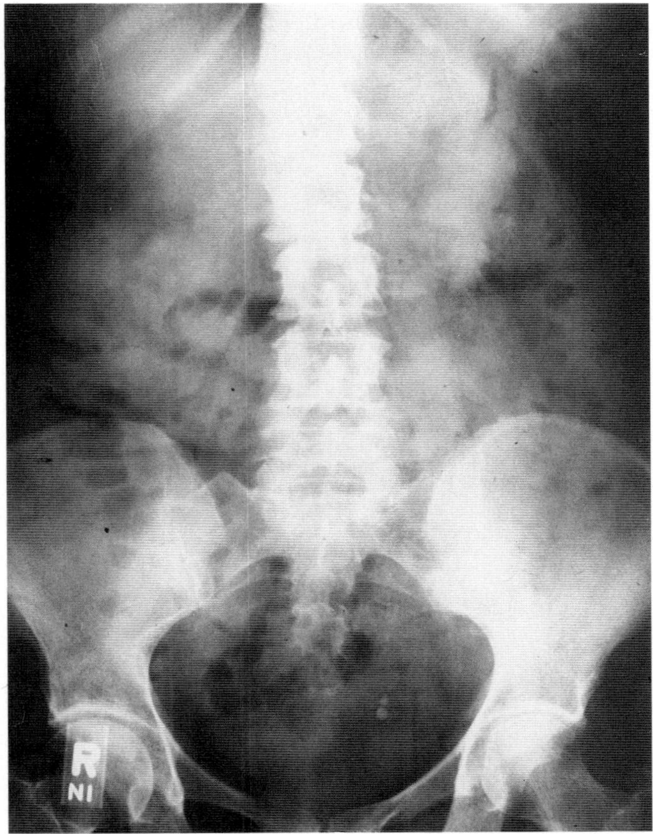

Fig. 123. Case 35. Scout film of the abdomen showing an abnormal axis of the right kidney and radiolucencies misinterpreted as bowel gas

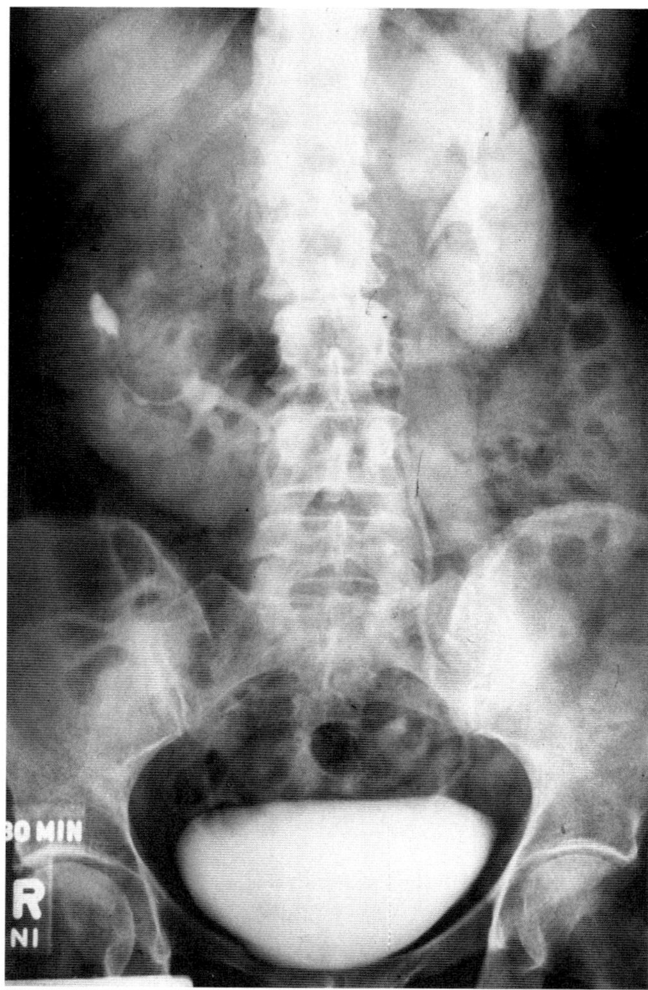

Fig. 124. Case 35. An excretory urogram reveals an infiltrating process affecting the pelvocalyceal system and extending beyond the kidney. Note lucent areas within the mass

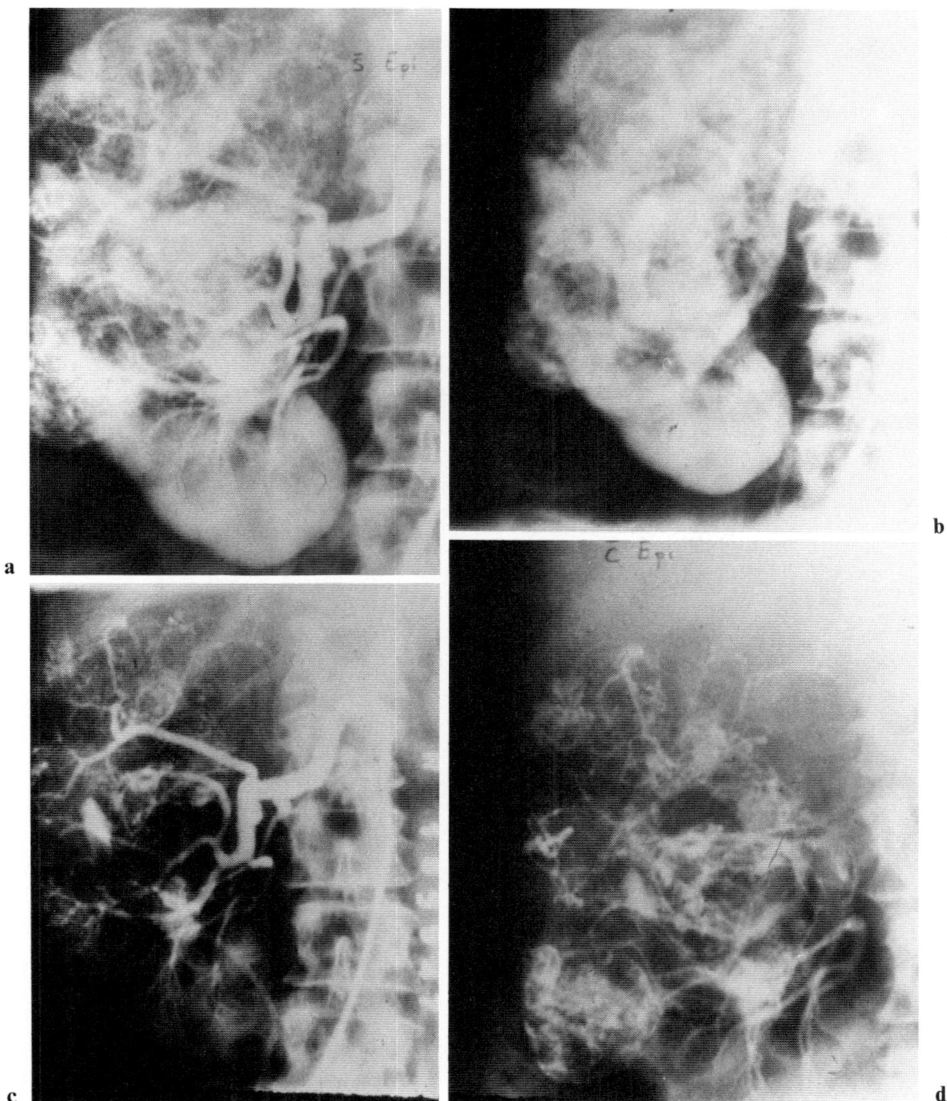

Fig. 125 a–d. Case 35. Arteriograms obtained without the injection of an arterial vasoconstrictor (**a, b**) and following the injection of epinephrine (**c, d**). Note extensive hypervascularity extending beyond the outline of the kidney. The vessels within the lesion fail to constrict (**c, d**). The diagnosis of an extensive carcinoma was made. At surgery, a carcinoma was suspected to be present. Histological section revealed an angiomyolipoma

The failure of lesions to exhibit vasoconstriction merely indicates the absence of receptors in the wall of the vessel. Lack of vasoconstriction can be seen not only in carcinomas but also in angiomyolipomas and in some infections.

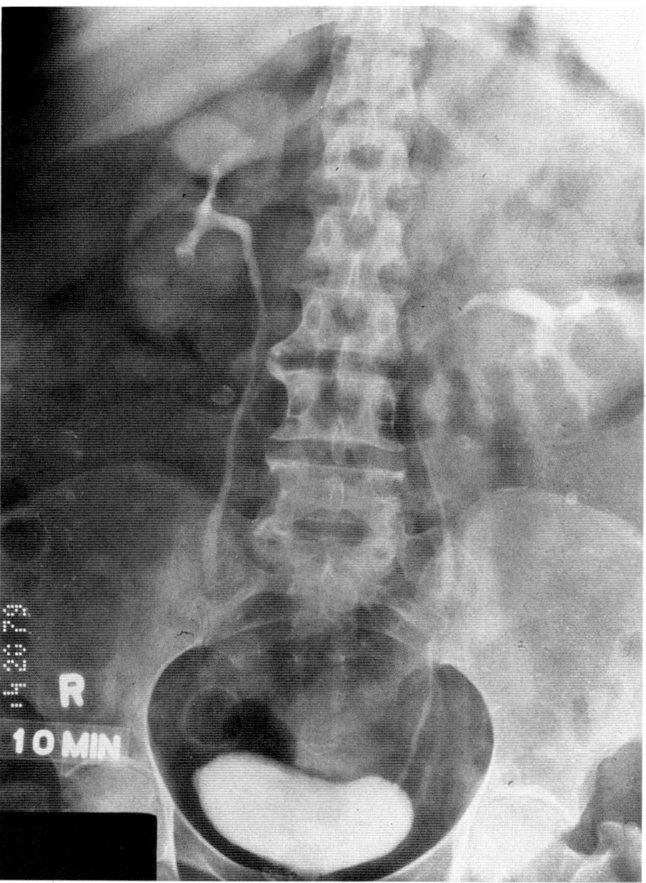

Fig. 126. Case 36. Urogram revealing a mass in the upper portion of the left kidney. Carcinoma of the left kidney was suspected

Fig. 128. Case 36. Selective left renal arteriogram showing minimal neovascularity within the mass. At surgery, this proved to be another angiomyolipoma

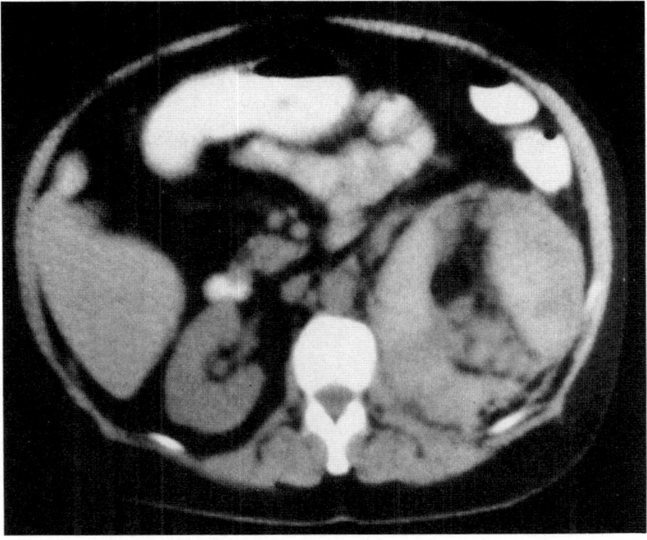

Fig. 127. Case 36. CT scan showing low density areas within the mass which correspond to fat

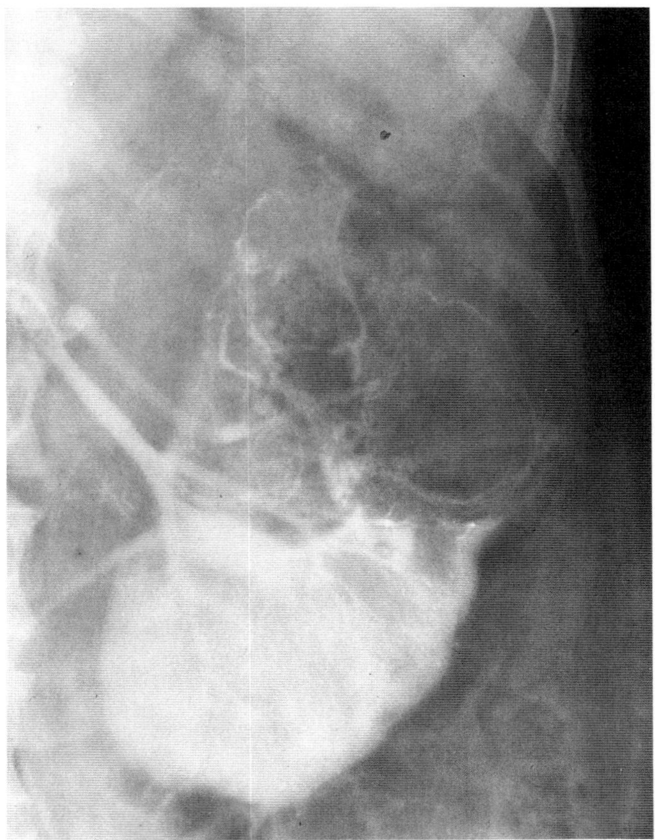

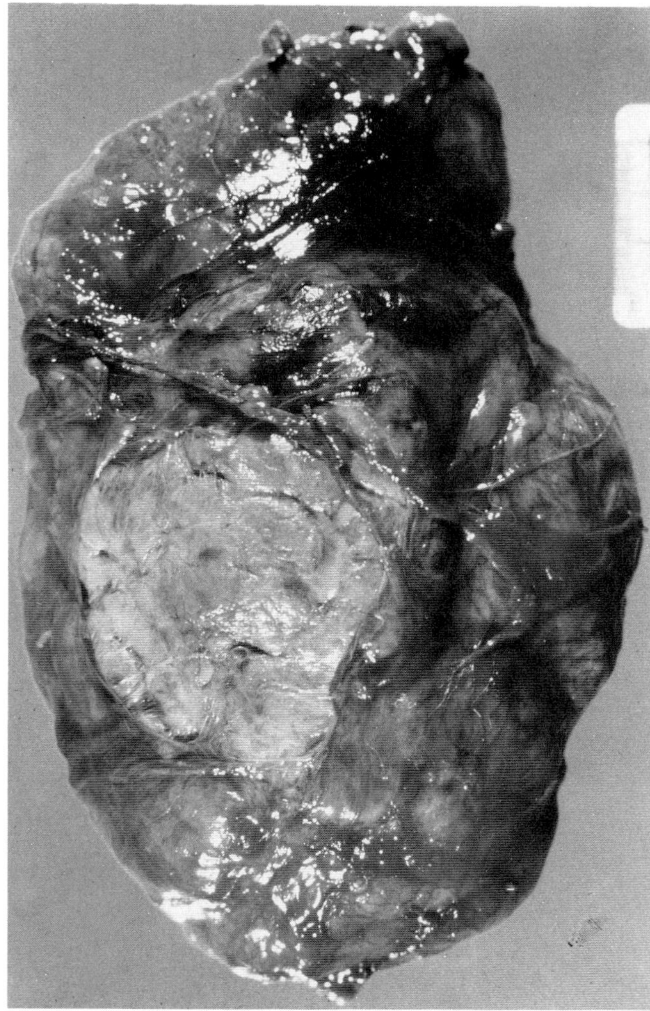

Fig. 129. Specimen of case 36. Clear area represents the abundant fat in this angiomyolipoma

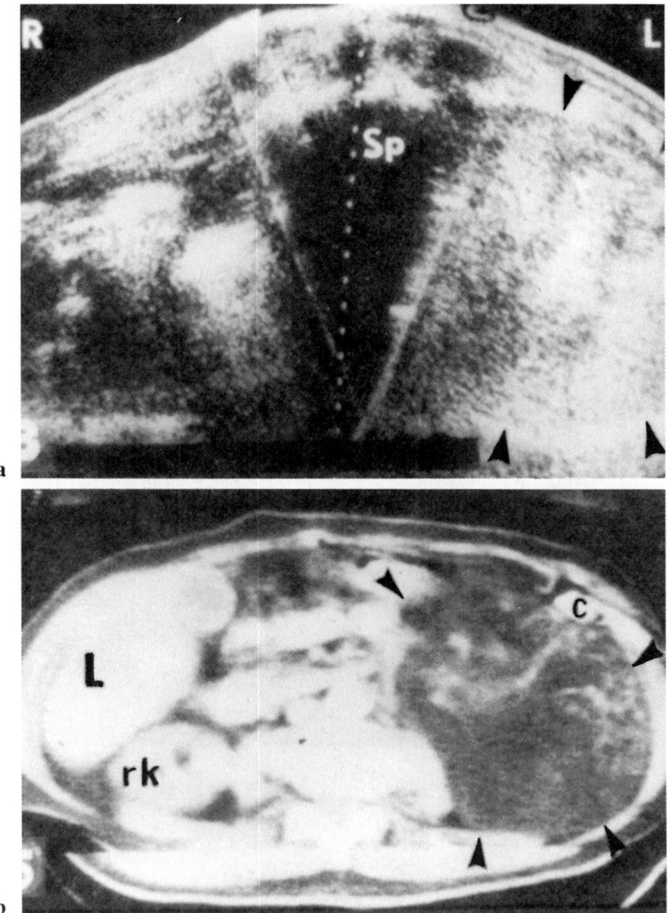

Fig. 130. a Ultrasound and **b** CT examinations in angiomyolipoma. Note the speckled echogenicity (*arrowheads*) throughout the lesion on the ultrasonogram. On the CT scan a mass is visualized (*arrowheads*) that had negative attenuation values, pathognomonic of fat. *Sp*, spine; *C*, cover of left kidney; *L*, liver; *rk*, right kidney

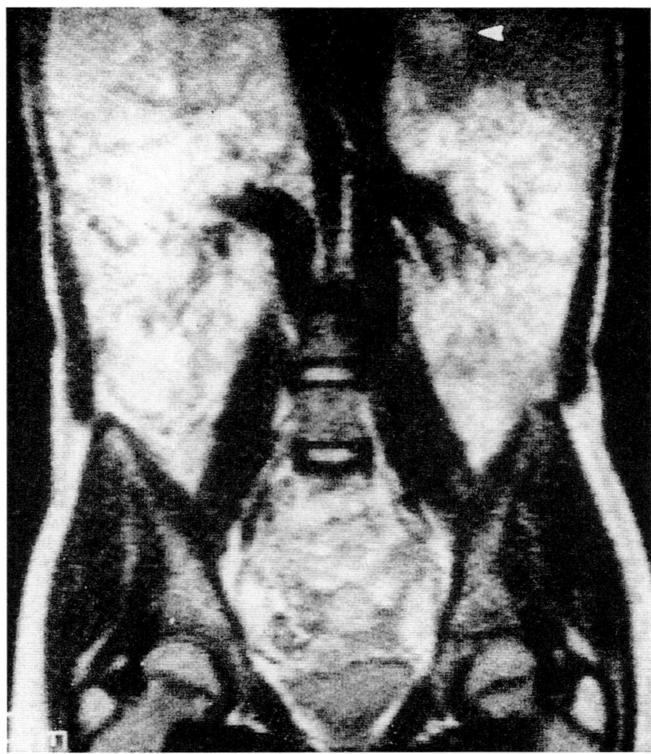

Fig. 131. MRI of angiomyolipoma in patient with tuberous sclerosis. Note the high signal produced by the fat within the lesions. A focal area of increased signal intensity of the upper pole of the left kidney (*arrowhead*) could be fat, normal parenchyma, angiomyoma or an associated tumor

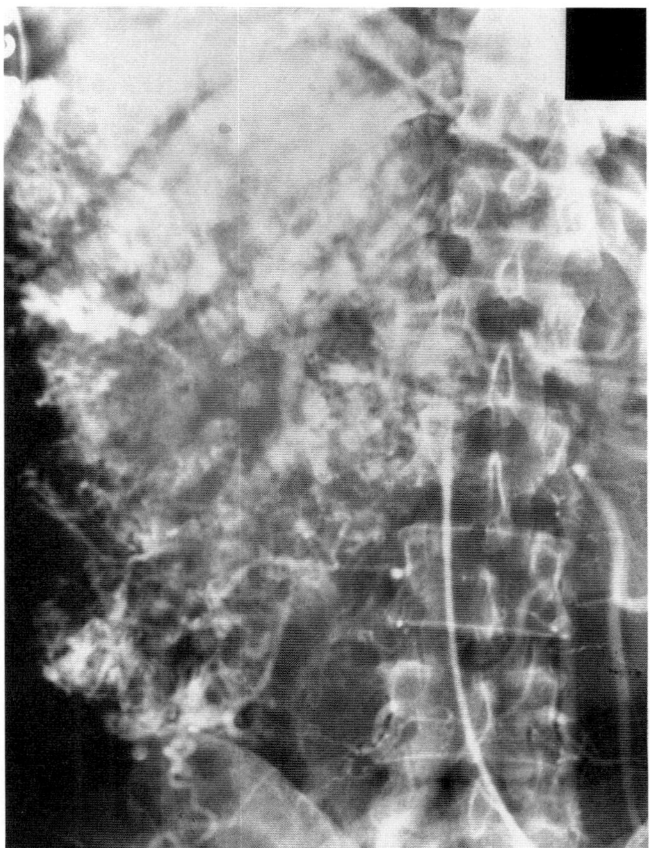

Fig. 132. Diffuse angiomyolipoma of the kidney. This angiogram shows hypervascularity of the tumor that extends beyond the kidney. Such lesions are prone to bleed and this is the most serious complication of angiomyolipomas

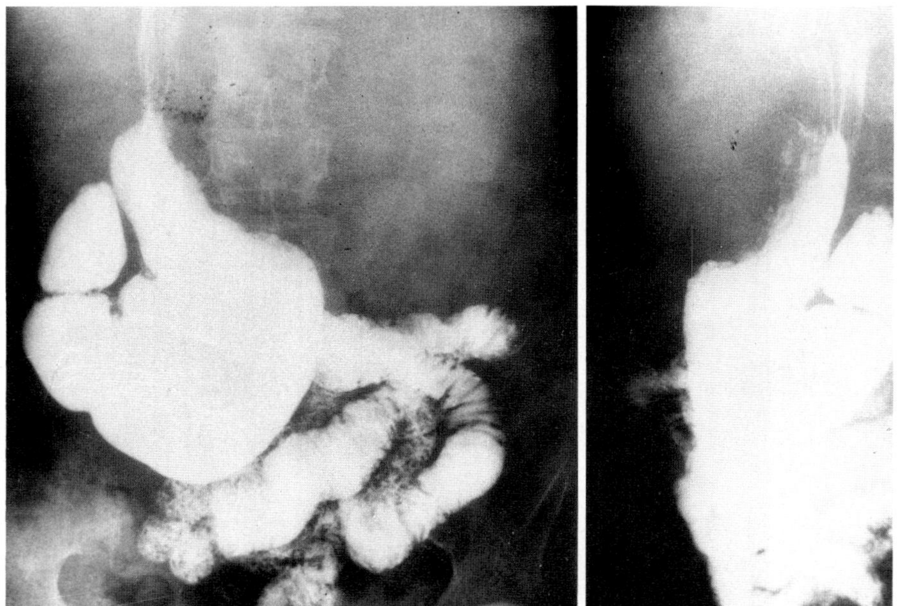

Fig. 133a, b. Case 37. Images from an upper gastroinestinal series (**a** frontal view; **b** lateral view). Note mass displacing to the right the stomach, which also appears to be displaced dorsally. Because of the dorsal displacement of the stomach, the diagnosis was an enlarged left lobe of the liver

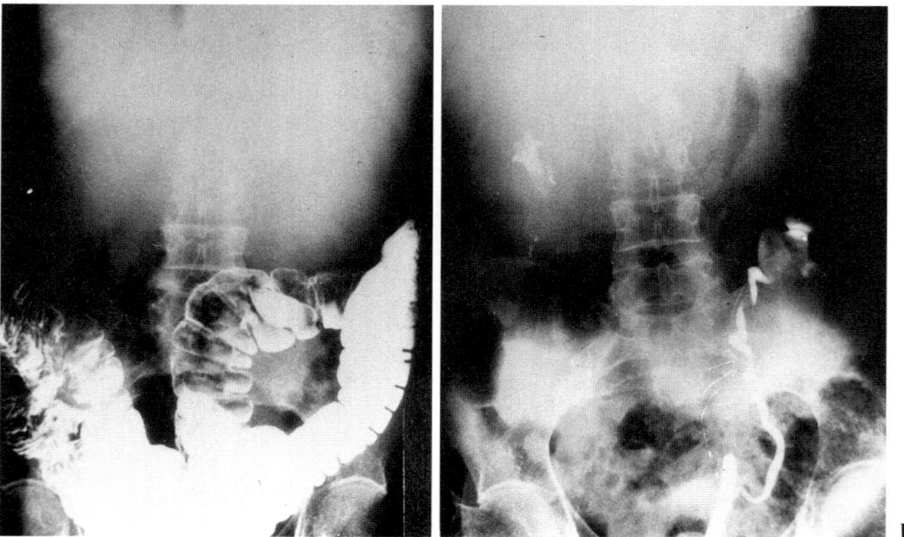

Fig. 134a, b. Case 37. **a** Barium enema study and **b** urogram. Note the downward displacement of the distal transverse colon and splenic flexure on the barium enema film, and also the downward displacement of the left kidney. This displacement should have suggested the retroperitoneal origin of the tumor

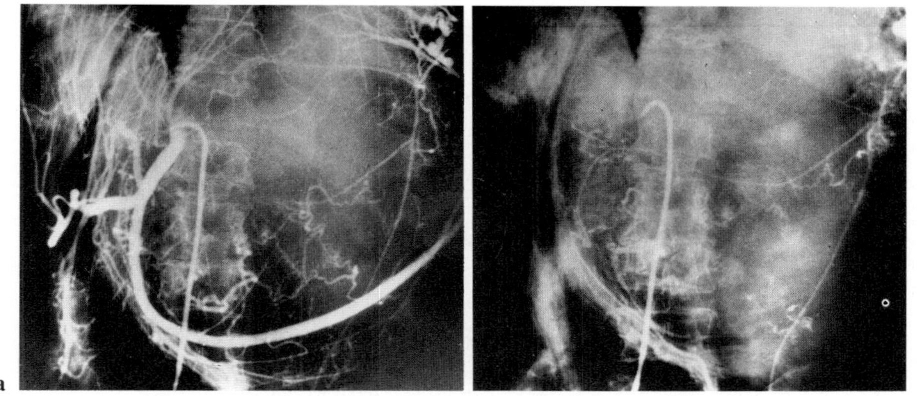

Fig. 135a, b. Case 37. Selective celiac arteriography, frontal projection. Note downward displacement of the splenic artery and neovascularity

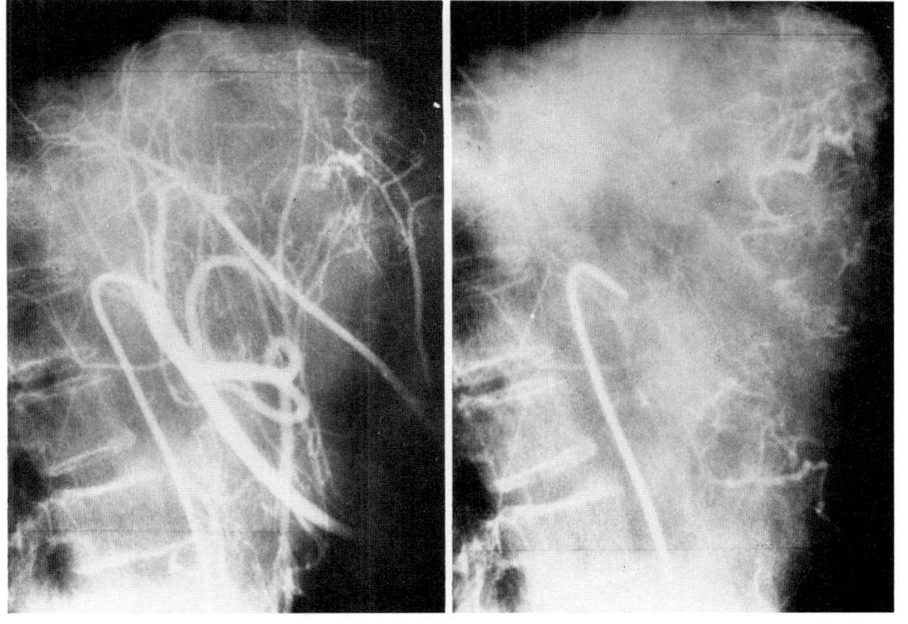

Fig. 136a, b. Case 37. Selective splenic arteriography, lateral projection. Note the large size of the mass extending from the retroperitoneum into the abdominal cavity. At surgery this proved to be an adrenal carcinoma

Some retroperitoneal tumors, by virtue of their massive growth, can displace intra-abdominal organs in an atypical fashion. Ventral growth of the tumor suggests the intraperitoneal origin of the neoplasm. Downward and/or medial displacement of the kidneys should suggest the retroperitoneal origin of the tumor

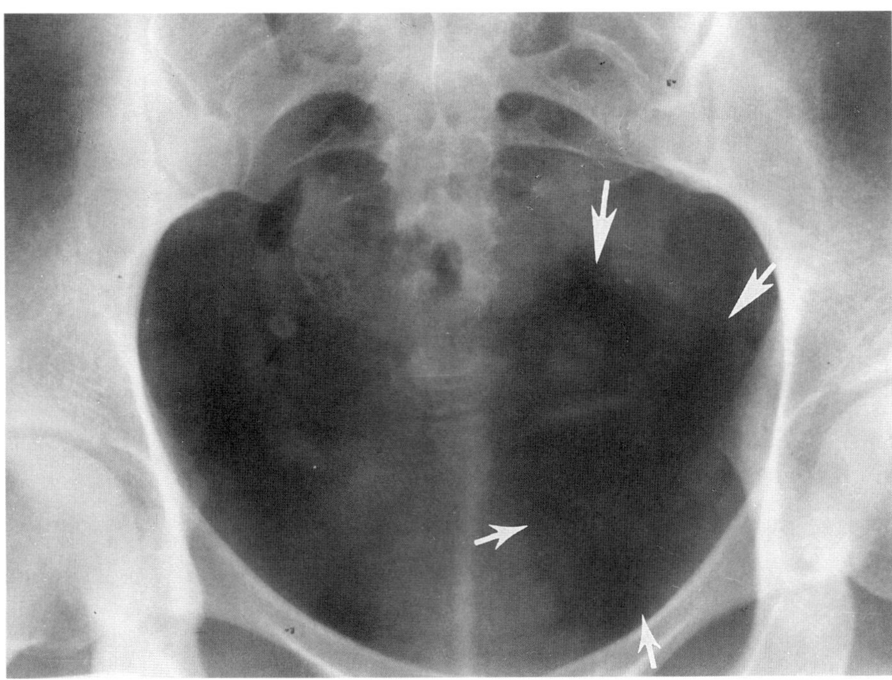

Fig. 137. Case 38. Lucency in the left side of the pelvis (*arrows*), which was thought to represent intestinal gas

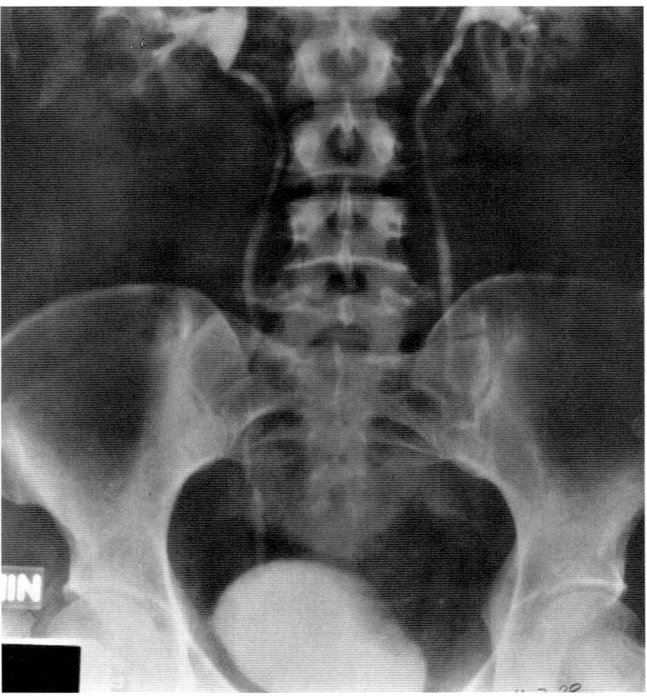

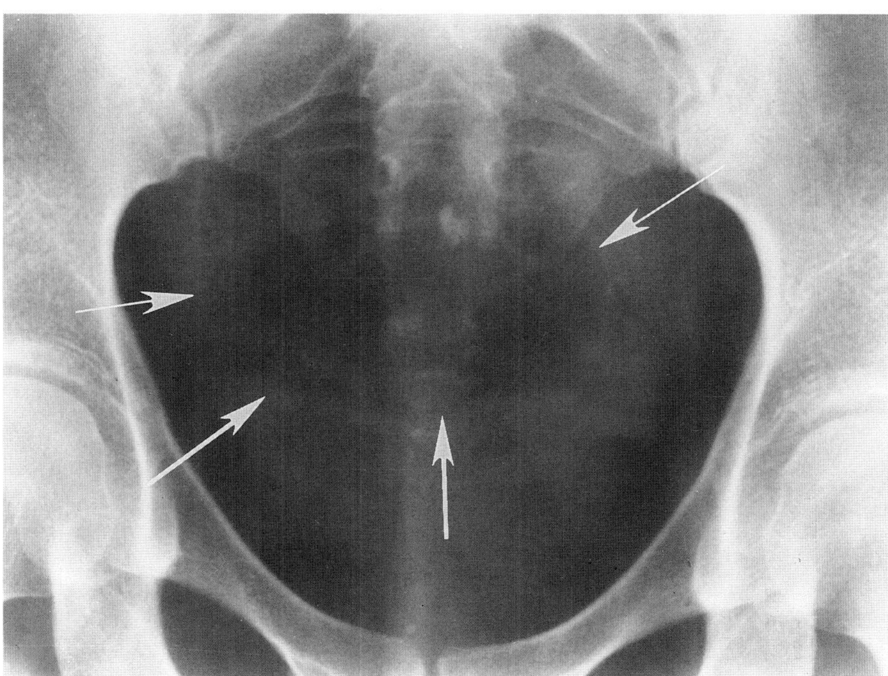

Fig. 139. Case 39. Film of the pelvis. Note radiolucency in the central portion of the pelvis above the urinary bladder (*arrows*). This also represented a dermoid. Occasionally, fat within the uterus can produce such radiolucencies

◄———

Fig. 138. Case 38. Urogram showing compression of the left side of the urinary bladder by a mass which is radiolucent. This finding is pathognomonic of a dermoid

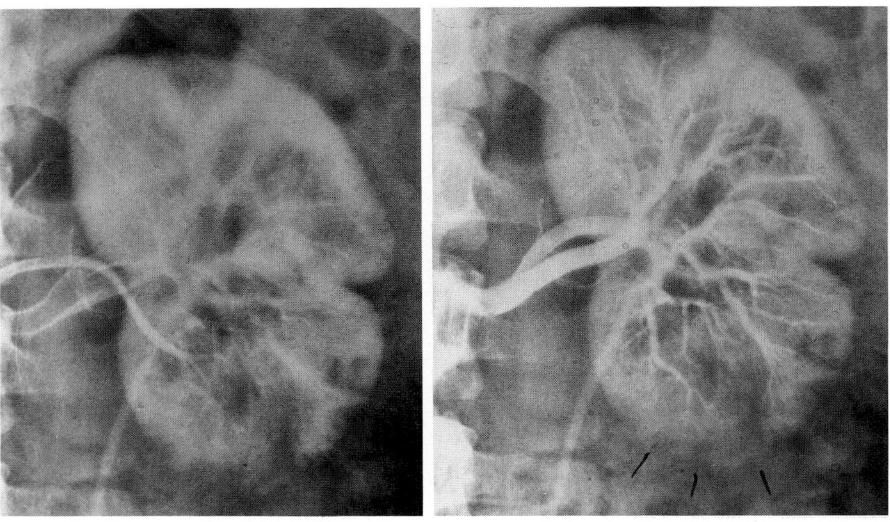

Fig. 140 a, b. Case 40. An error in interpretation due to poor technique. **a** Selective left renal arteriogram revealed an apparent defect in the lower pole of the left kidney. **b** Injection of accessory left renal artery showed that this area was supplied by the accessory artery and was intrinsically normal

When doing angiographic examination, if a selective angiogram fails to produce complete opacification of the organ, mid-stream aortography should be done in order to identify possible accessory renal arteries, which should then be selectively injected.

Finally, errors in diagnostic imaging can occur when physicians (nonradiologists) decide to study themselves in their own offices. I know of several physician-patients who have studied themselves using suboptimal equipment, often with an inadequate technique, and, most importantly, without thorough knowledge of how to interpret accurately the results of the diagnostic procedures. Often they have used the wrong diagnostic tests for the problem they had. These errors can easily result in poor management, the victim being the physician himself. I am now going to describe a sequence of errors which resulted from poor practice and probably caused the early demise of a dear classmate of mine.

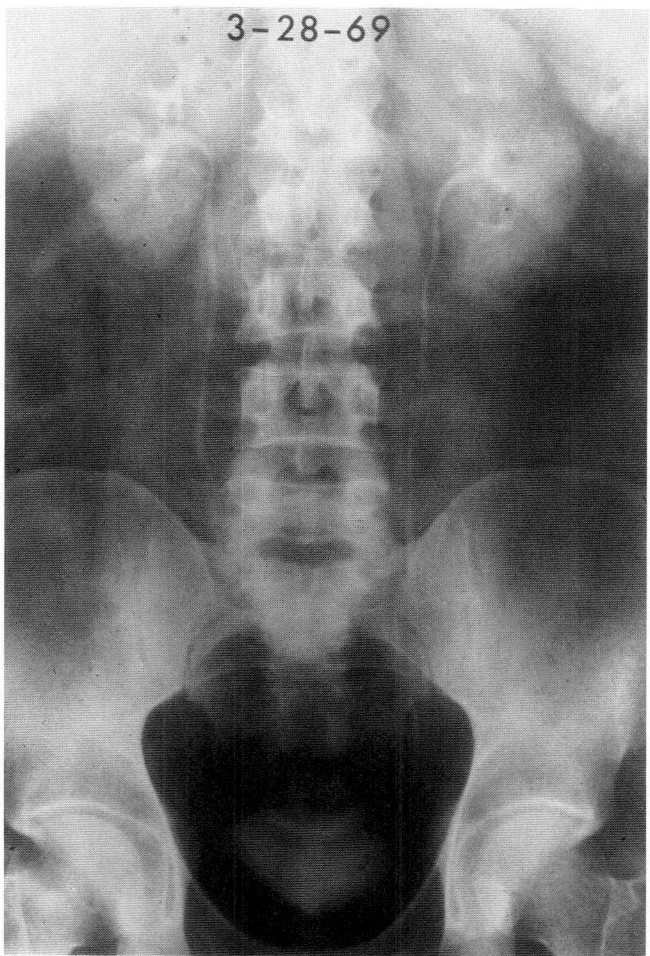

Fig. 141. Case 41. Dr. M.I.V., then aged 39, had right upper quadrant and right flank pain. He decided to have intravenous pyelography in his private office. This excretory urogram, dated 28 March 1969, was interpreted as negative. Technically it is a poor examination because the upper pole of the right kidney is not well demonstrated. Retrospectively, one can identify crowding of the right upper calyces

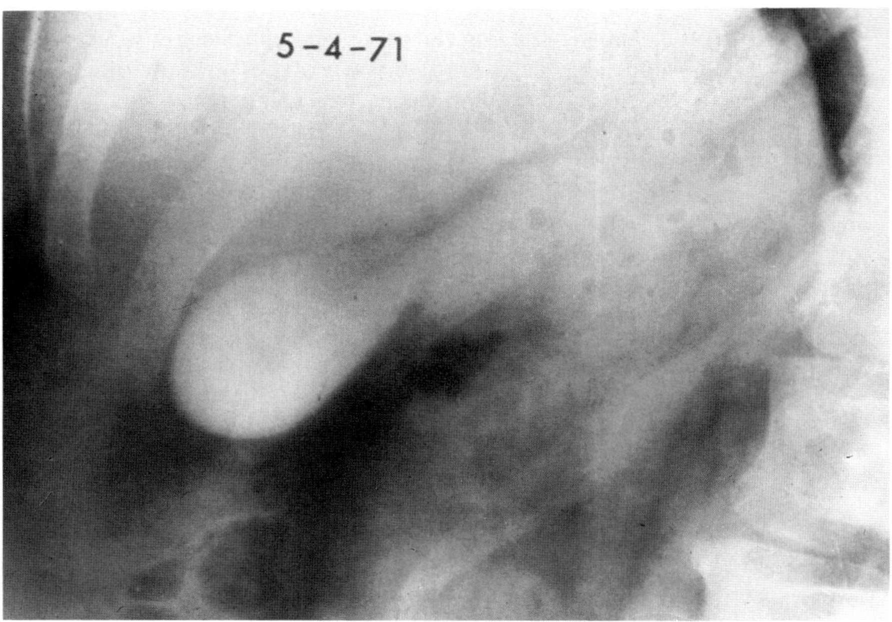

Fig. 142. Case 41. The pain continued intermittently, but he decided not to have any additional examination until 4 May 1971. This oral cholecystogram was also taken in his office. The gallbladder is radiographically normal, but the upper pole of the right kidney appears radiographically indistinct. This was not appreciated

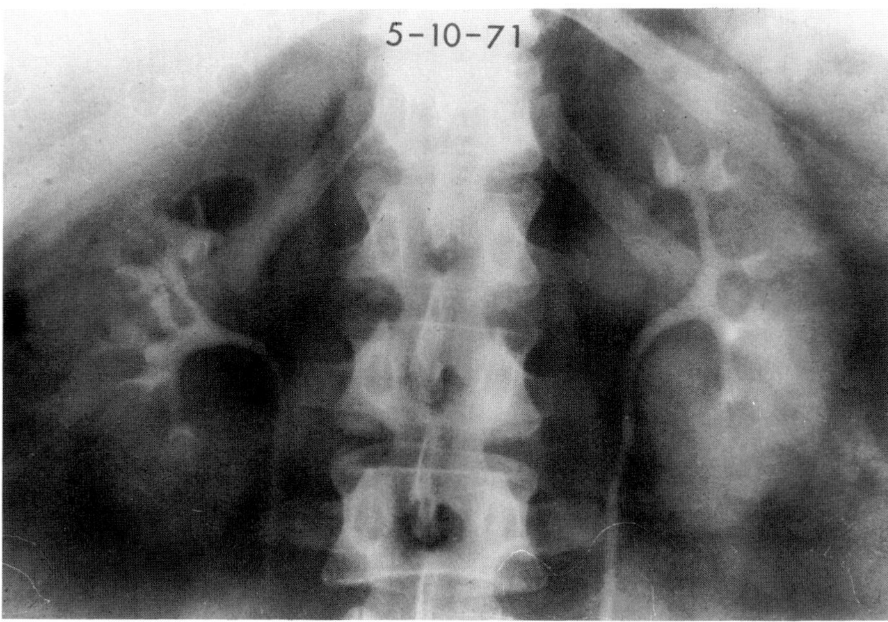

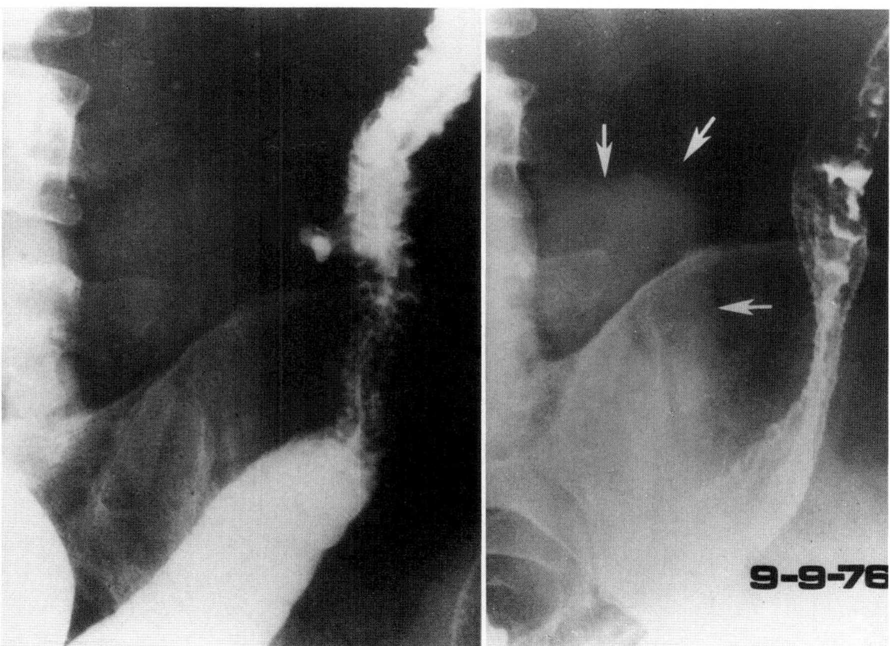

Fig. 144. Case 41. After surgery, the patient had no further complaints until September 1976, when there was left lower quadrant discomfort. This colon examination was ordered. Note a soft tissue mass to the left of the spine (*arrows*) and a diverticulum in the vicinity of this mass. The clinical impression at that time was of a "walled-off abscess from perforated colonic diverticulum." Additional investigations were performed as a result: ultrasound (Fig. 145), CT (Fig. 146), an isotope study (Fig. 147), and a repeat excretory urogram (Fig. 148)

◄

Fig. 143. Case 41. A week later, a repeat excretory urogram was performed. At this time, a mass was noted in the upper pole of the right kidney (note the indistinctness of the outline of the kidney and crowded calyces). An extensive renal carcinoma which had invaded the inferior vena cava was found at surgery. Despite several complications resulting from the surgery, the patient recovered

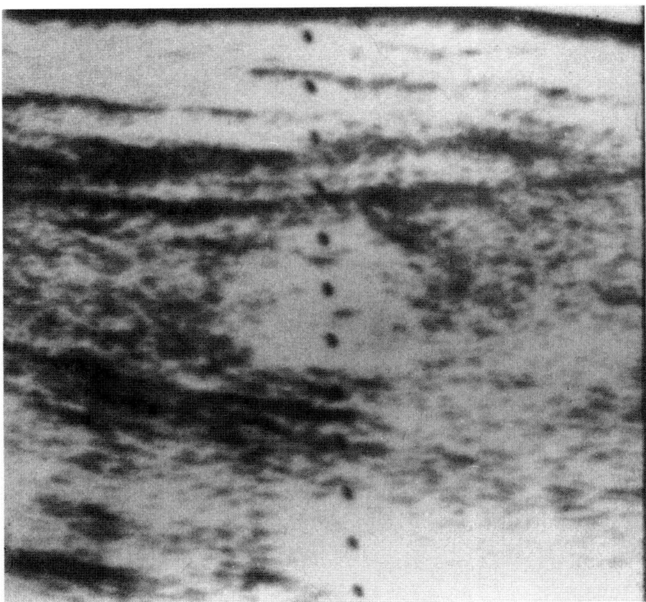

Fig. 145. Case 37. The sonogram revealed a well-circumscribed mass with internal echoes and slight posterior shadowing

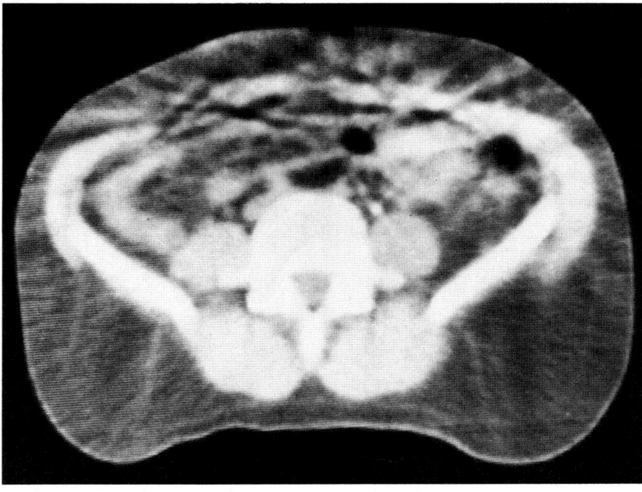

Fig. 146. Case 37. The enhanced CT examination revealed a left lower quadrant mass which appeared solid

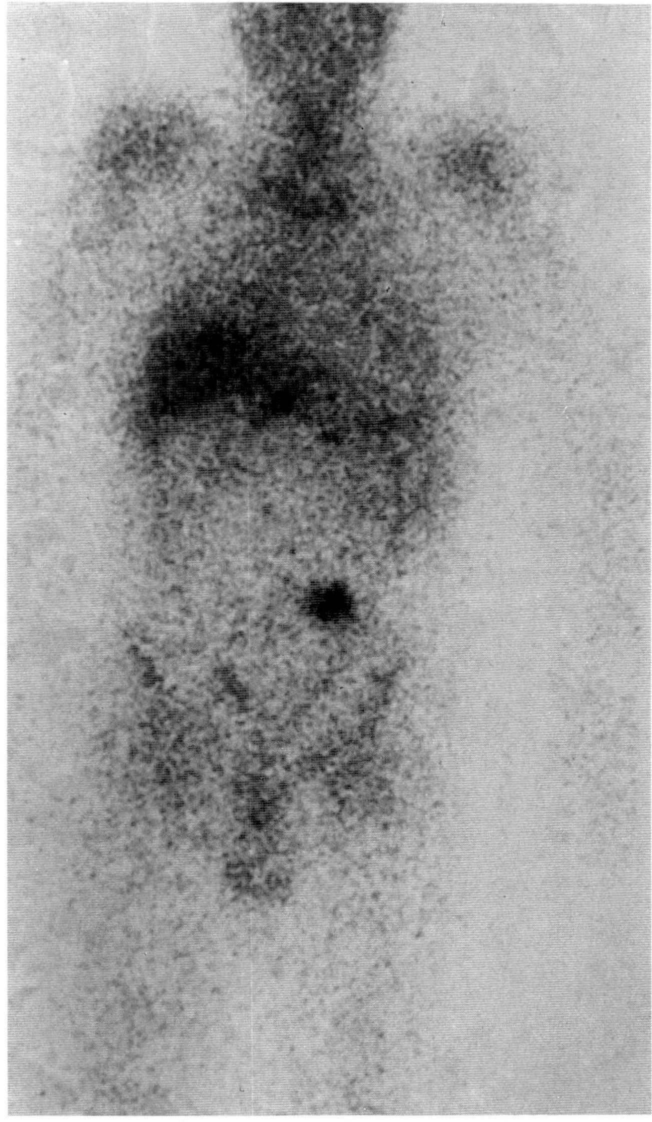

Fig. 147. Case 41. The gallium scan showed intense uptake at the level of the mass

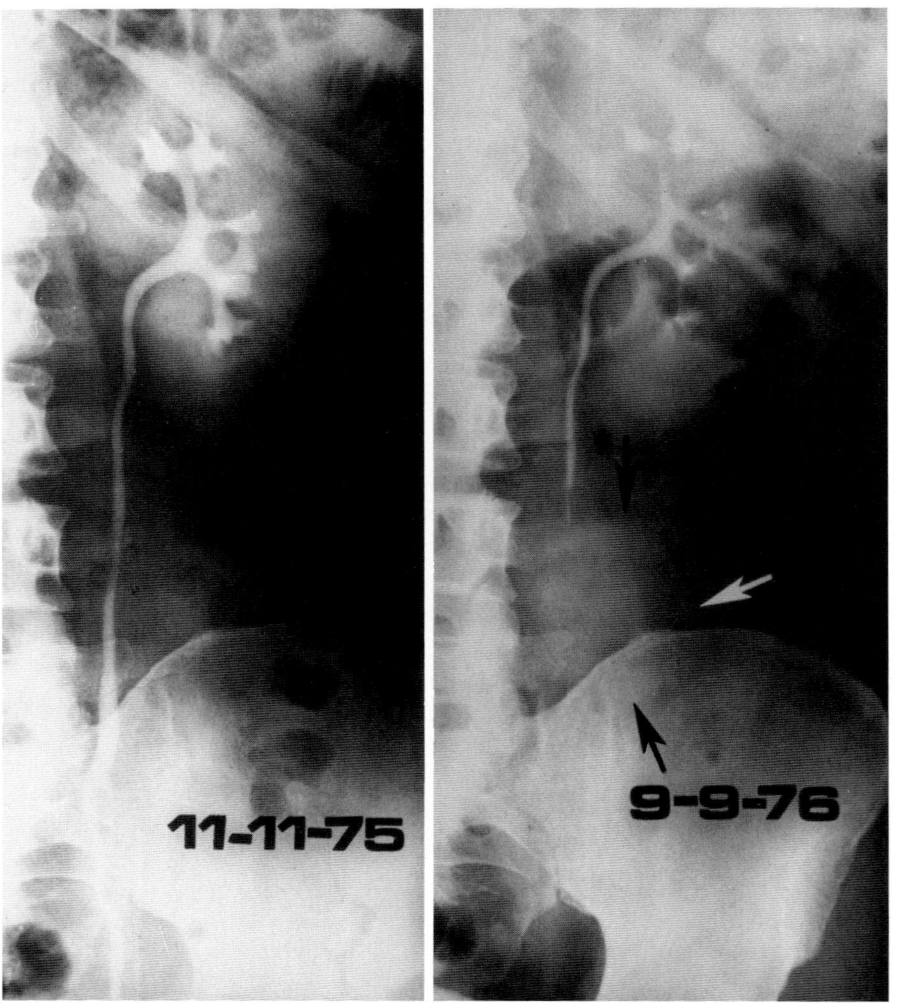

Fig. 148 a, b. Case 41. The repeat excretory urogram (**b**) taken on 9 September 1976, when compared to the one of 11 November 1975 (**a**) revealed that the mass was not related to the left urinary tract. My classmate was re-explored and a solitary metastasis to the mesentery was resected. Focal liver metastasis was found 2 years later (1978). In Houston, Texas, he underwent partial hepatectomy and developed respiratory distress syndrome immediately after surgery. This caused his death

Appendix: Tables

Table 1. Renal cystic diseases

1. Simple cyst (present 50% of individuals over 50 years of age)
2. Multilocular cyst (benign, multilocular, cystic nephroma)
3. Polycystic disease (infantile, adult)
4. Renal dysgenesis (multicystic disease, renal dysplasia, polycystic disease with abundant stroma)
5. Cystic disease of the renal medulla (medullary sponge kidney, medullary cystic disease)

Table 2. Synonyms for multilocular cystic nephroma

1. Benign multilocular cystic nephroma
2. Multilocular cyst of the kidney
3. Cystic nephroma
4. Cystic adenoma
5. Benign cystic differentiated nephroblastoma
6. Cystic nephroblastoma
7. Well-differentiated polycystic Wilms' tumor
8. Lymphangioma
9. Partially polycystic kidney

From: Madewell JE, Goldman SM, Davis CJ, Hartman DS, Feigin DS, Lichtenstein JE (1983) Multilocular cystic nephroma: a radiographic-pathologic correlation of 58 patients. Radiology 146: 309–321

Table 3. Radiologic findings in multilocular cystic nephroma

Technique	Findings
Plain radiography	Abdominal mass, occasionally with curvilinear calcification
Excretory urography	Well-defined intrarenal mass in a normally functioning kidney; occasionally internal linear densities (septa) are present; there may be growth into the perirenal space
Retrograde pyelography	Tumor herniation into the pelvis
Renal scan	Decreased excretion of radionuclides
Ultrasonography	Multiple circumscribed sonolucent areas separated by intense echoes
Computed tomography	Large, smooth, multiloculated mass; septa enhance with intravenous contrast; locules do not enhance
Angiography	The tumor is usually hypovascular, although it may be avascular or hypervascular
Cyst puncture	Clear yellow fluid; filling of locules directly punctured

M. Viamonte Jr.,
Mount Sinai Medical Center,
Miami Beach, FL

Errors in Abdominal Radiology

1992. IX, 91 pp. 50 figs. in 176 sep. illus. 6 tabs.
Softcover ISBN 3-540-54080-6

Why are mistakes made in abdominal radiology? In this book, a companion volume to his book on errors in chest radiography, Dr. Viamonte explains how many errors are caused simply by wrong techniques or faulty interpretation. How can a specialist avoid making such mistakes? By recognizing the reasons for past mistakes.

The author has collected many such cases during thirty years of experience, which he discusses with regard to the liver, spleen, and pancreas, the hollow viscus of the alimentary tract, and the retroperitoneum.

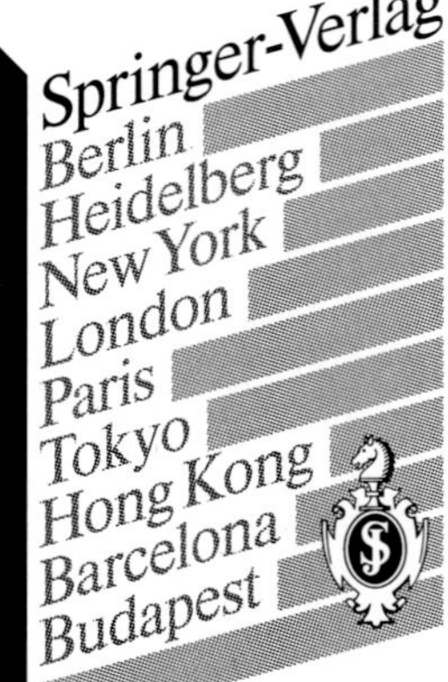